*"This gives us confiden*

*help our son achieve whatever he desires,*

*as long as we teach him the discipline*

*he will need to overcome this*

*obstacle in his life."*

*"I think that it is super*

*that you try to create a greater awareness*

*of diabetes.  As always, you are proving*

*to be a leader, not only on the field,*

*but off the field as well."*

*"I just wanted to thank you*

*for being such a good role model for me."*

*Cover photo of Jay Leeuwenburg courtesy of Roche Diagnostics*

# Yes I Can! Yes You Can!

## TACKLE DIABETES AND WIN!

**DENNY DRESSMAN**
AND
**JAY LEEUWENBURG**

**COMSERV BOOKS**
LLC

DENVER

Copyright © 2005
Denny Dressman and Jay Leeuwenburg

All rights reserved.
No part of this book may be reproduced in any form
or by any means without permission in writing from the author,
except for brief quotations embodied in critical articles and reviews.

For information, contact
ComServ Books
P.O. Box 3116
Greenwood Village, CO  80155-3116
www.YesICanYesYouCan.com

Yes I Can! Yes You Can! Tackle Diabetes and Win!
LCCN: 2005935623
ISBN: 0-9774283-0-3

Production Management by
Paros Press
1551 Larimer Street, Suite 1301     Denver, CO 80202
303-893-3332     www.parospress.com

Book Design by Scott Johnson

Printed in the United States of America
1  3  5  7  9  10  8  6  4  2

*For Erika and Rachel.*
*May God bless you with Jay's determination,*
*in pursuit of every goal you set*
*and in the face of whatever adversity*
*life may hold for you.*

D.D.

*To Ingher, my life coach and partner.*
*I would not have reached such heights*
*or become half the man I am without your*
*love, strength and insight.*

*For my daughters, Cora and Kate Louise.*
*May I inspire you both to be anything you want to be,*
*and to always have hope in your hearts.*

J.L.

# PROLOGUE

THE NORTHERN Coast of Oregon, like most of the state's Pacific Ocean shoreline, is one endless public beach, filled with postcard scenes and travel guide features.

For decades families have come to the beach houses and campgrounds to spend their weekends, holidays and vacations in an area where green forest and rocky cliffs meet wide sandy beaches, rolling dunes and windblown ocean waves.

It's a place where countless and varied birds soar over the cliffs and skim the ocean's surface, perch on the huge rocks nearby or scurry along the beach, always just ahead of the next incoming wave.

It's a place sea lions and other marine animals call home, where vacationers can go crabbing and fishing boats return from the deep sea with their catch, and where lighthouses stand silent sentry.

Altogether, it's a most unlikely place for a young boy to come face-to-face with the hard reality of his future.

Yet here, in the land of high-flying kites and quiet coves, Jay Leeuwenburg's life changed in a way neither he nor his parents could have imagined, and which at first not even the doctors could explain.

For a while, they feared he was dying. He had just turned 12.

*We were going to Oregon on vacation to stay at the beach house my grandfather built. It's in a small community named Manzanita, which is about 15-20 miles north of Tillamook, where they make the Tillamook Cheese that's sold in stores all over the country.*

*On the flight to Portland, I drank all the orange juice they had on the plane. The flight attendants were saying, 'Wow, you have a growing boy.' But that's not what it was. I had an unquenchable thirst.*

*I look back on that now, and I realize the signs were there a couple weeks earlier. It was a family tradition that we'd always go canoeing on rivers in Missouri in the summer. We had a cooler with two cases of soda for five children and four adults. I drank every soda.*

*I had been urinating a lot, but I thought that was because I drank so much. Then I started losing weight. I went from around 150 to about 115 in three weeks! I'd lost 36 pounds in less than a month — when I was supposed to be hitting a growth spurt.*

*I had what I now know are all the classic symptoms, right down to my breath. My mom was always complaining that my breath stank. She said I wasn't brushing my teeth. But it was the ketones. If you spill what are called ketones, it essentially means your body can't use all that sugar.*

*In Oregon, I was dehydrated. I was throwing up and hallucinating. I was there to have a good time, and I didn't even know where I was. My family had no idea what was going on. Meanwhile, I kept feeling worse and worse.*

*They took me to the community clinic in Wheeler, another little town near Manzanita. They tested me for mono, and didn't find a thing. They were stumped. A day or two later, my dad took me to a hospital in Astoria.*

*When I finally found out that I had Type 1 diabetes, my first reaction was, 'Good, I'm not going to die.' That was a real concern because neither my parents nor I had any idea what was going on. It was very scary.*

*I felt extremely relieved knowing that this was something that was treatable. I understood almost right away that it would change my life – without comprehending what that meant. But it wasn't cancer, and it wasn't something that would be immediately life-threatening. I would start feeling better. I would be able to continue to go to school.*

*From my first breath after finding out I had diabetes, my first question was, 'Will I still be able to play sports?' I made that a priority.*

*At 12, I had no idea what would happen to my athletic career. I certainly wasn't thinking about being a pro football player. I hadn't even played a minute of organized football by the time I was entering eighth grade.*

But I was already a very active and competitive person. I was playing soccer, basketball, church softball; I swam all the time. I'd go for a bike ride for three hours; I literally rode my bike for three hours. Neighbors would see me riding, a long way from home, and they'd stop and ask me if everything was all right. Or I'd hit tennis balls against a wall for hours, or shoot baskets. I'd always be doing something athletic.

Minus anything else happening to me, I refused to not be able to participate. I had to be able to play any sport I wanted. I needed that physical outlet.

They said I would be able to, but I'd have to make some modifications.

# CHAPTER 1

# A DIABETIC FAMILY

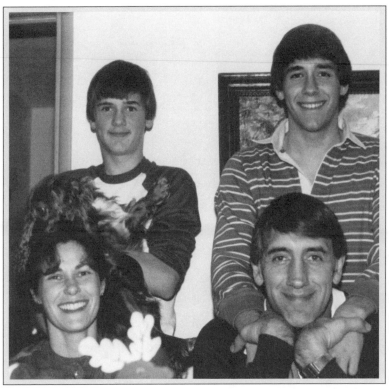

*Photo courtesy of Dick and Jann Leeuwenburg*

*"From the get-go," explains Jay's brother Chris,
"we were really immersed in it as a family.
It was a lifestyle. We knew, to be successful,
it was something you did as a family."*

WALKS ON the beach were a part of every vacation trip to Oregon for Dick and Jann Leeuwenburg. But those relaxing, leisurely strolls took on a different character the summer the younger of their two sons was hospitalized for treatment of his newly diagnosed diabetes.

Jay's older brother Chris, a high school sophomore at the time, saw a side of his dad he didn't know existed.

"It was the most vulnerable I'd ever seen my dad," he recalls. "It really broke him up. My dad's a big guy, 6-feet-5. He played pro football. Growing up, I thought he was pretty tough. But when we found out Jay had diabetes, I'd never seen him so emotional."

As they trudged through the sand, Dick and Jann wrestled with the emotions, questions and fears that torment all parents as they come to grips with the news that their daughter or son has developed a chronic, incurable illness that could blind, cripple and kill her or, in this case, him.

First came the feeling that they were responsible.

"We talked a lot, and we cried," Jann says. "We both felt guilty, like you did something to your child. Guilt is not rational, but it's there nonetheless."

Jann wracked her brain for clues from previous generations of her family and Dick's. She wanted to know: How could this happen? Could they have done something to prevent it? Should they somehow have known there was an increased risk?

"My mother was gluten-intolerant," she says, "which is definitely a pre-cursor to juvenile diabetes. When she was an infant in 1918 she spent a year in a hospital. Dick has auto-immune diseases on his side of the family."

Quickly they began to second-guess their responses, or rather their initial lack of any response, to Jay's out-of-character symptoms.

"Once it's diagnosed," Dick says, "you think, 'Boy, were we stupid! How big did that billboard have to be before we saw it?'"

"It's terrible to admit all the things you did wrong," Jann chimes in as she relives the experience from memory. "We were at a friend's house on the beach when Jay threw up. The day before we had taken him to the little clinic nearby, and had him tested for mononucleosis. And he of course came up negative for mono. But they didn't catch the fact that he had acetone breath and all of these classic symptoms.

"The next day, when Jay started vomiting again, that's when Dick said, 'Something's wrong. I'm taking you to the hospital.' I think it scared Dick more than me. I didn't even go with them."

Dick Leeuwenburg doesn't remember the name of the doctor who examined Jay at Columbia Hospital in Astoria that day, but he remains impressed with the physician's immediate recognition of Jay's problem.

"We sat down with the doctor and told him what was going on, and he called the nurse and had her take Jay right out for some tests. Then he said to me, 'We'll have those tests, but I'll tell you what they're going to tell us. They're going to tell us your son has diabetes.' He didn't need any tests; they were just something he had to do.

"I didn't even know what diabetes was," Dick admits. "I knew the word, but I didn't know what the heck it was. I knew diabetics took shots because I'd actually roomed with a diabetic when I played professional football.

"I was in training camp with Pittsburgh, and I was rooming with another lineman who was trying to make the team. I don't even remember his name. But I remember there was insulin on the room air conditioner to keep it cool, which is how I knew he was diabetic. But that was the total extent of my knowledge.

"Looking back on it, had we been alert, we would have known well before we got to Oregon that summer. Once you understand the symptoms, it's hard to miss them."

When they talk about signs that should have been hard to miss, everyone in the family mentions the canoe trip that preceded the vacation in Oregon. Looking back, Jay's brother now realizes that what was happening was far from normal.

"We went on this canoe trip every year with a couple of other families. The summer Jay was diagnosed, five of us rode in our family's station wagon. One of the neighbor's sons, who was in college, drove our car. It was Jay, me, John and his two sisters.

"It was a four-and-a-half-hour drive, and we were stopping all the time. We had to pull over, it seemed like every few miles, because Jay had to pee. And he was always thirsty. Everybody was giving him a hard time; the girls gave him the most trouble."

A BLOOD SUGAR reading measures the milligrams per liter of sugar in the blood, and a normal reading ranges from 70 to 120. Jay's on the day his dad took him to the hospital was almost 950.

Jay's tests didn't take long. When he returned, the doctor surprised Dick, though not with the diagnosis.

"Jay needs to hospitalized," he announced.

"Oh, okay," Dick answered, figuring he meant a stay that might wait until the family returned to St. Louis. "When?"

"Right now," the doctor said.

"I was stunned," Dick recalls, "but it was obvious to anyone who knew Jay. He was always bouncing off the walls. But he had no energy. He was listless, a 90-year-old man inside a kid's body."

Dick went from stunned to amazed a few minutes later when he witnessed, first-hand, insulin's dramatic impact on the human body.

"While I'm filling out the papers for him to be admitted to the hospital, they gave him his first insulin shot. It was immediate, like flipping a switch: Jay's back!"

Dick recalls Jay "taking over" Columbia Hospital almost

immediately after being admitted.

"He owned that hospital. You'd go in there to see him, but Jay's not in his room. He's over in the physical therapy wing, and he's off riding their bicycle. They wouldn't let him out of the hospital, so he had to make do with what was in the hospital."

*I was only in the hospital three days. But in three days, they taught me about the juggling act between insulin, food and exercise.*

*When you are diabetic, Type 1, your body does not produce insulin. The function of insulin is to convert sugar into useable energy for your muscles.*

*Everything you eat is broken down into sugar. That sugar is in your blood stream, and it needs a way to get into the muscles. That's what insulin does. It's the key that unlocks the door to let that sugar get into your muscles.*

*The balance is finding out how much insulin your body needs to convert that sugar into energy. That's where it's tricky; every body is different.*

*And when you exercise, you use a greater amount of sugar. If you burn a lot of sugar while you're exercising, you can have too much insulin in your body. Then you need more food so that insulin has something to work on. That's the juggling act.*

*What you eat influences how quickly things are digested, and turned into sugar. The times for these digestive conversions are called glycemic indexes. Fats take the longest to break down. You eat a high-fat meal, and you're not going to get a sugar spike. Protein is the next slowest, then complex carbohydrates like natural grains and fibers, whole fruits. Those take longer to be broken down, but they're still much quicker than proteins. Then comes simple and processed sugars. Soda is processed. It's almost instantly absorbed into your blood-stream.*

*Without insulin, you have all that sugar flowing around your blood-stream that can't be used efficiently by your muscles. That's not just your quadriceps and your biceps. It's your heart, your lungs, your brain, your eyes – all those things that people don't associate with "muscles". If your blood sugar is too high, you can go into a coma.*

*A low blood sugar reading means the body has too much insulin. There's not enough sugar to feed on. Insulin is going to work whether you have sugar in your blood or not. Insulin with no sugar starts breaking down muscles in the body – your body almost cannibalizes itself.*

*And guess what "muscle" is easiest to break down. The brain. That's why diabetics pass out and can go into a coma when they have extreme or prolonged low blood sugar.*

*When I was diagnosed they didn't use calorie counting to manage the juggling act. They used a system of exchanges. A slice of bread is one carbohydrate exchange. A quarter cup of cooked rice is a carbohydrate exchange. A whole banana was two carbos.*

*Part of our education was meeting with a dietician. I remember my parents having to measure everything until they got used to what exchanges were. You learn a lot more about food.*

*I remember asking, "Why is mayonnaise a fat?" And saying, "I don't know what an artichoke is. I know it tastes good, but is it a vegetable? Is it a starch?" Corn is not considered a vegetable. It's considered a starch.*

*My dad loves ice cream. Typically he would have a bowl of ice cream after dinner about half of the time. So we would have discussions at dinner. He'd say, "I'm going to have ice cream, so you better not eat that dinner roll if you're going to have ice cream with me, because that's a carbo for two fats." We would have conversations about the choices you made, and how that was going to affect what you eat.*

*Kids today don't have to understand exchanges. Now they count carb grams. You can find this number on the label of every package. Kids with diabetes don't gain an understanding of diet the way you do if you have to learn exchanges.*

WHILE JAY was learning his first lessons in how to take charge of his diabetes, his mom was learning to how to give him his insulin injections, and how to respond to the signs of extreme low blood sugar.

"I remember when Jay was diagnosed, thinking, 'Oh, my! Jay has to get shots.

"I got a syringe and some saline solution, and practiced

giving shots to a grapefruit. The doctors and nursing staff said that was as close as you were going to get to human skin, the feel and the texture, and the way the needle would go in. So I spent half a day giving shots to a grapefruit.

"I was very scared about Jay getting a low blood sugar, particularly with his high energy level and activity. That's when I would get really nervous. Would he learn the signs and be able to treat it quickly enough?"

Potentially catastrophic low sugars are treated with what is called a glycogen kit. It's essentially a super-loaded sugar shot. It is administered to diabetics only in emergencies, when they get so low they refuse to eat and get incoherent or belligerent.

"You mix a liquid into a vial that creates this syrup," Jann explains. "Then you draw it into this syringe and you inject it into the diabetic. The preferred spot is into the butt – through the clothes if you have to.

"I practiced, even if I wasn't going to be giving Jay any regular insulin shots. I had it in the back of my mind that I needed to feel relatively comfortable, because it would likely be me giving him that glycogen shot if he ever needed one. As it turned out, I never gave Jay a shot of any kind."

It was Jay himself who liberated his parents from their anxieties and self-doubts, during another walk on the beach after he returned from his three days at the hospital. It was typical Jay.

"Chris, had to get back home for the start of football practice," Jann recalls, "and Dick had to get back to work. So they went back to St. Louis together while Jay and I stayed with my parents for another week or two just so Jay could get accustomed to the phenomenon. And so he could have some vacation. He hadn't really had any vacation because he spent the whole time sick and in the hospital.

"I remember walking on the beach one day after he was diagnosed, and he told me at one point during our walk, 'Mom, I had a talk with myself.' He said he told himself, 'Hey, I can accept this and get on with my life, or I can fight it, and say, 'This isn't happening to me, and woe is me.'

"And he told me he just made a personal resolve, right then and there, to get on with his life, which I think is a phenomenal thing for a 12-year-old to do.

"But that's Jay. I'm sure he was frightened, but he wasn't teary or clinging. He just wasn't a dependent person."

*What was really beneficial for me is I was old enough to understand what was happening to my body. Now, kids can be diagnosed as early as six months old. They have no clue why they're being poked with these needles. They don't know what insulin is.*

*I was extremely fortunate that I could ask some questions and comprehend the answers. I wanted to take responsibility and say, 'I understand. If I don't take this, I'm going to die.'*

*I was able to say, 'This is something I'm going to have to live with for the rest of my life, so let me start out by doing it.' In my opinion, that was a really important* step I took instantly, because I knew it was something I had to control.

My mom and dad came to the realization very quickly that it didn't matter what they did, they could not "fix" my problem. The comment they'd get from other parents was, "Thank goodness Jay will take his shots. Because so-and-so's little boy or little girl didn't take his or her shots, or never took their blood sugars. Just feel lucky that Jay's actually taking care of himself."

One of the big apprehensions about having diabetes is having to give yourself injections of insulin. That can be very difficult for many patients.

It just so happened that the guy in my room when I was admitted was in for rabies. With rabies you have to use extremely long syringes and give yourself a shot in the stomach. I think, either from the suggestion of the doctors or maybe because he wanted to try to help me, he went out of his way to say, 'Hey, listen, look at what I have to do. I can tell you this hurts.'

In comparison my syringe was so little, and the amount I had to inject was so little. It actually made it so much easier. This guy, who was probably somewhere in his 30s, had probably been scraped or bitten by some cat or dog, and he didn't even know if he had rabies. But he had to take these shots for a week anyway. To know that, it didn't seem so bad that I had to take these little itty-bitty shots.

THE CHALLENGE facing the Leeuwenburgs was to become what Jay calls "a diabetic family." That means encouraging a single, healthy lifestyle for everyone, and resisting the inclination to make allowances or to treat that child differently. It is one of the most important steps the young and newly diagnosed diabetic's parents and siblings must take.

There were several things about the Leeuwenburg home that gave them all a head start on meeting this challenge. Eating meals together had always been a priority. The expectation that the boys would apply themselves in school and make something of themselves was as clear as could be. And both already had that competitive fire.

"From the get-go, we were really immersed in it as a family," Jay's brother explains. "It was a lifestyle. We knew the alternative was really bad. We knew, to be successful, it was something you did as a family.

"Jay fully embraced what he had to do," Chris says. "That's the way our family always was. There weren't a lot of excuses for things. There wasn't an option of doing anything else.

"We knew if we wanted to play sports in high school, we had to keep our grades at least at a 3.0. And we always knew we were going to go to college and get a degree, because that was the expectation."

Chris attended Purdue University then became a Wal-Mart store manager. It was as an adult that he saw what can happen without the kind of influence that was present when he and Jay were growing up.

"I've actually worked with a lot of diabetics in my adult

life, and it just makes me have that much more respect for my brother. It was an excuse for a lot of them. They're giving into it. I guess they didn't have the support group to see it as a challenge rather than as a disability.

"That's unfortunate, because it was never looked on that way in our house. It was never, 'Take it easy on Jay.' "

It wasn't that Dick and Jann ever took Jay's illness lightly or forgot about it. They just learned to cope.

"You have to get past the low-level stuff," Dick explains. "Somebody says diabetes, and you start learning about it. There are all these unhappy outcomes out there, and they're always there.

"We didn't get preoccupied with those kinds of negative things. But it was never so far back in your mind that you forgot about it. It's still there, but it just blends in."

Adds Jann: "You have your life, and then you have that other awareness."

*My mom made our family a diabetic family. She didn't ever say, "Here's Jay's meal, and this is for everyone else." It was never, "Sure, Chris, you can have this, but Jay, you can't."*

*My mother has always been health conscious. Even before diabetes we would ask her, so what's the latest health kick? So after I was diagnosed, it was always, "This is healthy living, and this is going to be our lifestyle."*

*She never made me feel I was a burden. I didn't*

understand and appreciate this until I was older. I would
have recognized it if it had been the other way.

One of the values that I still subscribe to with my family
is that we sit down to the dinner table as a family, every night,
no exceptions. That was a priority when I was growing up.
We would hold dinner sometimes until 7 o'clock until dad got
home from work, because that was the expectation.

We always ate breakfast together as a family, and we
always ate dinner together as a family, even before I was
diagnosed. That's important to point out because, for many
people with diabetes, eating the same things at the same
time as the rest of their family is a huge lifestyle change.

It didn't have as much impact on our family as on
others. Meals were always a positive focal point for our
family structure. That's when we would always have
family talks and reflect upon the day. We always had
engaging conversations.

One time our dinner table topic was saccharin, the
artificial sugar, because I needed to limit my sugar. We
were discussing a study that said it caused cancer in lab
rats, and my dad said, "Well, hell, if you feed rats enough
oranges, that'll give them cancer, too. If you give lab rats
enough of anything, even if it's good for you, it'll probably
cause cancer at some point."

My dad is very caring, but in a reserved kind of way.
There's no doubt there was an overwhelming love from my
mother and father, but he didn't talk about it much. The
exception is that he was comfortable giving hugs.

*Besides being Mr. Unemotional, my dad is very analytical. He did not want me to feel like I was being treated like a baby. He wanted me to cope with these issues and deal with them. His whole attitude was, it didn't matter if I was a diabetic or a kid dealing with the peer pressure of alcohol and drugs, or with making bad choices, this was my life and I needed to live it.*

*My dad didn't expect me to be perfect with diabetes, but he expected me to learn from my mistakes. It's part of growing up, to learn from your mistakes. He likes to use the analogy that they were going to give me rope to lean out over the edge, but not enough to hang myself, and just enough that if I leaned too far over that cliff, they could pull me back.*

JANN LEEUWENBURG is an accomplished artist whose work is regularly on exhibition in a gallery in Manzanita. Before she developed her talent as a painter, she was an elementary school teacher. Growing up, she says, she was a free spirit whose body matured well before her mind.

Ever the more serious and practical sort, Dick is what you would expect of an economist. He enjoyed a successful business career in executive management after his brief taste of pro football.

Recalling their second son's childhood in a continuing stream of simultaneous right-brain/left-brain recollections, they jointly paint a vivid portrait of the irrepressible youngster who ultimately overcame longer odds than usual in becoming an elite professional athlete.

"Jay wasn't that 'pity me, let's see what I can get out of this, how much emotion I can get out of people to use to my advantage' kind of kid," Dick explains.

"Nobody has ever given Jay a shot but Jay," Jann quickly adds. "Except that first shot he got in the hospital," Dick clarifies. What they don't say is how rare it is for 12-year-olds to administer their own injections.

"Jay's always been a 'take-charge-of-my-life' kind of person," Jann recalls with amusement, "not always looking to me for permission to do what he wanted to do." ("Sometimes unfortunately," Dick offers, still with a hint of fatherly disapproval almost 30 years later.)

"Jay was in nursery school," Jann resumes, "and one day I got a call from the teacher, Mrs. Durbin. 'I just wanted to let you know that Jay decided he didn't want to be in school today, and apparently he's walking home.' It's at least a mile and a half, and he's walking home! I went looking for him and picked him up along the way. But that was just Jay.

"You didn't dress Jay," she goes on. "He would get up in the morning, and would put on outlandish outfits, but he had a clear vision of what he wanted to wear." ("He'd come down to breakfast," Dick picks up, "and I'd go, 'What in the world do you have on?' It was just what he wanted to wear that day.")

"It was delightful to me, in a way," Jann smiles fondly. "I didn't want to interfere with it.

"One of my favorite stories about Jay is from right before we moved a few blocks from where we were living in Kirkwood, a St. Louis suburb. He was in the third grade, and he had a pogo stick. He decided – He set his own goal for himself; it was nobody's idea but his – that he was going to ride his pogo stick from our new house to our old house. "It was maybe a half-mile. And this was without missing. If you fell off, you had to start all over again. He did that for an entire summer, but by God, he did it! I think he even got over there, and then came back without missing."

At this points Dick jumps in. "This was a non-trivial exercise. It was hard to do, crossing streets and going up and down hills. You just go, 'There's Jay.' It wasn't really that far out. It was in keeping. Maybe it kind of pushed out a bulge on one edge, but it wasn't a free-standing, 'Where did that come from?' kind of thing for Jay."

"It was just his personality," Jann offers. "I have to say, it is a trait that I really admire: the ability to set a goal and just be hell-bent on accomplishing it."

*I would always put goals out there for myself that didn't necessarily have a rhyme or a reason. There was a time I decided I was going to ride my bike to a place 25 miles away, just to go that far on my bike. I was determined I was going to do it. And so I did it.*

*When I got this pogo stick, I wasn't very good at it, at first. It was something you needed some coordination and some athleticism to do, and it didn't come to me instantly easily.*

*So I wasn't content with doing it just okay. I had to*

be the best at it. So it seemed logical: Why not pogo stick
a half-mile, or however long it was? I didn't think of it as
any major accomplishment. It was just that I set my mind
to it. It took me a while, but I did it.

   The route is ingrained in my mind. You had to go
down the road on Dickson, and then there was this street
called Crescent, and you went up the hill. It split in two,
and you went to the left, and down a big old hill. Then you
crossed a very busy street called Woodlawn. You cross
Woodlawn, and Crescent becomes Bodley. And then you go
up Bodley – one, two, three houses on the left. Our house
was three houses up Bodley on the left.

   Just a little further up Bodley was another big hill,
and I decided that was the place to learn to ride my bike no-
handed. That's the way I was. Many times I was an all-or-
nothing kind of guy.

   I was determined I was going to ride my bike no-
handed. I couldn't do it when I was going slow. So I said,
where's the biggest hill I can think of? So I went to the big
hill up the street, and pedaled that bike as fast as I could. I
didn't figure on the front tire wobbling like it did. I still
have scars on my knee to prove it.

   My left knee went on the pavement for about three
feet. I left my bike in the middle of the street, and hobbled
to our house. My mom put me in the kitchen sink and took
one of those little scrub brushes and scrubbed all the rocks
out of my knee. Then she put a Band-Aid on it and said,
'You're good.'

# CHAPTER 2

# 'DIABET-OLOGIST'

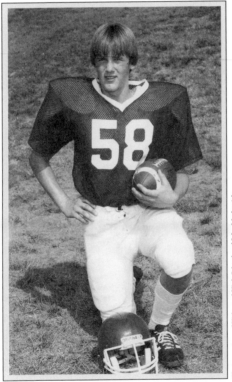

Photo courtesy of Kirkwood High School and John Markovick

*"Give me the tools and I'll use them,"*
*Jay told his doctor. "Because it was never*
*an option to not play. That would have been*
*like saying, 'You can't breathe.'"*

WHEN THE LEEUWENBURGS moved that half-mile pogo stick hop from East Bodley to Dickson, a prominent St. Louis orthopedic surgeon, Dr. Perry Schoenecker, became one of their new neighbors. As soon as Jay was admitted to Columbia Hospital, Dr. P, as Jay and Chris came to call him, was the person to whom Dick Leeuwenburg immediately turned for help.

"Somewhere in that day when Jay went to the hospital, the doctor there said, 'You have to get Jay hooked up with an endocrinologist,'" Dick recalls. "I called Perry right away.

"He said he'd take care of it. He called around, got references and interviewed a list of candidates. Then he called us in Oregon and told us, 'Here's who I think is best.' That's how Jay wound up becoming a patient of Dr. Pat Wolff.

"We got on the phone with her right away from Oregon. The first thing she said was, 'I'd like to talk to Jay.' She said, 'Just so you understand: I'll be Jay's doctor, not your doctor.'

"That was unexpected, but one of the things that tempered

how we reacted to this was that she wasn't a shot in the dark. You have someone like our neighbor tell you that, in his opinion and in the opinion of the area's medical community, she's number one in this field, and immediately she has a lot of credibility.

"The whole conversation had to do with things that made sense. Jay's the one who was going to have to manage it for the rest of his life, not us, so he ought to just start right now."

*There's a part of me that wants to believe the fate aspect of it. We put a bid on the house they lived in, but they had just purchased it. My mom and dad looked around, and two weeks later decided to buy the house next door. We were neighbors for ten years.*

*My brother and I called him Dr. P, for Perry. He was a very accomplished orthopedic surgeon, but he was very approachable and very congenial. I never had to call him 'Doctor' Schoenecker. If we didn't call him Dr. P, it was Mr. Schoenecker.*

*Chris and I played with his sons, and I remember they had a big poodle dog that we always played with. Theirs was the only house in the neighborhood that had a pool. Dr. P and his wife Sally were always very open to us coming over and swimming.*

*He is not the kind of guy who goes around calling in favors all the time. It's just not his normal practice; he takes his profession very seriously. So when he calls and says, 'I need a favor,' it's a highly unusual request and other doctors know it's important.*

*Having a next door neighbor like that, one who
wound up getting me treated by Dr. Wolff out of all the
doctors in St. Louis, seems like more than luck to me.*

PATRICIA B. WOLFF, M.D., was one of the most respected pediatric
endocrinologists in St. Louis for the last quarter of the twentieth
century. Yet as the New Millennium approached, and a new calling dawned with it, she stopped taking new diabetic patients.

"When you're caring for a diabetic," she explains, "it's
really a 24-7 kind of responsibility. It's impossible to provide
that kind of care if you're not here. I can't leave the country if
I'm doing that."

As a child Dr. Wolff had imagined helping the poor of the
world, but she did not realize her dream until she had married,
established her pediatric practice in St. Louis and was well into
raising a family.

She had worked a couple of years with the Indian Health
Service in Rapid City, South Dakota after graduating from the
University of Minnesota School of Medicine in 1972. But it was
not until 1988, when she visited Haiti for the first time, that she
began  actively to pursue her humanitarian calling. By then Jay
was into his second year at the University of Colorado.

Dr. Wolff returned to Haiti many times after that, working
in a church-sponsored clinic. In 2000, she took a sabbatical from
her private practice at Forest Park Pediatrics and from her position on the staff of St. Louis Children's Hospital and her teach-

ing responsibilities at Washington University in St. Louis to volunteer around the world. She has treated the poor of Uganda, Malawi, Cambodia, Honduras, Nicaragua and, always, Haiti, where the poverty is the worst she has ever seen.

In 2003 she established a program in Haiti she calls "Food and Meds for Kids." Its centerpiece is a malnutrition program that provides starving children 175 calories a day in peanut butter, sugar, oil, powdered milk, vitamins and minerals for each kilo of their body weight. It's a program she saw employed successfully by a colleague working in Malawi, an obscure and impoverished little country near South Africa.

Her passion was apparent in an article about her efforts in *Outlook*, a publication of the Washington University in St. Louis School of Medicine. "These are children who are barely alive, very lethargic, with orange hair," she said. "Then you see them six weeks later, and they are running around with chubby cheeks and new black hair. They look terrific by comparison."

Such a visionary physician was the perfect match for Jay, the indomitable adolescent, when they met in the late summer of 1981.

"He was very compliant, for a teenager, with what he needed to do," Dr. Wolff says warmly. It is clear from the tone in her voice that Jay was, and remains, a special case for her.

"He was very smart. That whole family was very smart. The more usual way is for the child, or really for anyone, even an adult, to be noncompliant, to be depressed and kind of like, give up. It makes them depressed to think they have to do all these things, and so they don't do all of them.

"To have a person just accept the fact they have this, and it's a problem to be managed, is quite rare. Most people spend their time emoting about it rather than managing it. When you come across a rational person, it's a sight to see."

*I often think about my mom and dad, and think this disease was harder on them than on me. I think they had some long, hard talks about how they could help Jay, and some sleepless and restless nights. As a young kid who thinks he's invincible anyway, I just looked at it as, 'This is the hand I was dealt, I'm going to make the best of it.'*

*It wouldn't have mattered if it was diabetes or something else. The values I was brought up with applied to this: You stay positive, find the best in any situation, work hard, and seek knowledge to make your choices the best you can make at the time. I still do that today.*

*Dr. Wolff set the tone at the beginning when she told my mom and dad, 'This is your son's disease. As much as you want to help him, he has to take responsibility for it."*

*I've seen countless times when the doctor doesn't tell the parents, "You know what, you can't live your diabetic's life for them." That was the right way for me and my family at the time. I was old enough to understand it, and take responsibility for it. She took something that could be extremely negative, and made it extremely positive.*

*The message was, "You're old enough to take responsibility, and that's what I expect as your doctor."*

WHAT JAY recalls as the turning point so early in his relationship with Dr. Wolff was in her mind an inevitable step.

"His parents, like many parents who are intelligent and well-informed but very fearful about the ultimate outcome, in their own anxiety wind up driving their kid crazy. The kid is getting resistant because the parents get overly controlling. It destroys their whole relationship.

"Their child has been rescued, and they've been told something about insulin and food and shots, but they don't really know what they're doing. The crisis of the coma is over, and the child is upright and walking. But how long, they wonder, will it be before he slips into another coma, or they give him too much insulin, or not enough. The child is less terrified because he's a child; it's the parents who really are terrified.

"All of a sudden they feel they have to be in charge of everything about their child's life. As you can imagine, the child resists that. The best way out of that is to make the child responsible for the problem.

"I perceived this to be happening with Jay; mom is saying one thing and the child is moaning and groaning. The next time they came in, I just told them, 'I'm going to have your mom wait outside.' "

Dr. Wolff's bottom-line message to Jay was a simple one.

"I told him, 'It's up to you. You're smart and you get this. We need to make a plan. When we have a plan, we'll call your mom in and tell her about it.'

"This relieves the parents from the feeling that they're responsible. Parents know they can't do it, but they don't know

who will do it if they don't. Jay said he was going to do it, and
he did it."


> *When I told Dr. Wolff that I wanted to be able to*
> *participate in sports just like any other boy my age, she*
> *said, 'I hear you loud and clear. But if you do that, I'm*
> *going to have to educate you on how you can do it success-*
> *fully, how you can do it safely.'*
> *My reaction was, 'Great! Give me the tools and I'll*
> *use them.' Because it was never an option to not play. That*
> *would have been like saying, 'You can't breathe.'*
> *Through the guidance of Dr. Wolff, I learned you*
> *need to be acutely aware of the signs your body is sending;*
> *what your body is telling you. Because athletically, that's*
> *how you get in trouble, if you don't pay attention to your*
> *body's signs.*
> *If you get a low blood sugar, and your brain starts not*
> *thinking rationally and you're exercising, that's when you*
> *can pass out, go into insulin reaction, then diabetic coma.*
> *Not only is it scary, it can be life-threatening.*
> *Even when I was playing in the back yard – Frisbee or*
> *hide-and-seek – I needed to be aware of the signs of having low*
> *blood sugar. Looking back on it, recognizing and listening to*
> *my body from an early age has served me well athletically. I*
> *was in tune with my body much earlier than my peers.*
> *Dr. Wolff told me I had to be able to feel the changes*
> *in my body when I was having low blood sugar. She told*

*me to choose an activity, and do that activity with a friend. She told me to have emergency food nearby. Basically, it was just 'run around until you start feeling goofy.' Then she wanted me to stop, take a blood sugar and verify that I was having low blood sugar, then identify how I was feeling. The first sign for me was I would feel extremely hungry. I'd be in a basketball game and feel like I needed to go to dinner.*

*Over time, I came to recognize other symptoms: shortness of breath, my recovery wasn't as fast as it used to be; it would be harder for my eyes to focus on smaller text. In the NFL, for example, we'd study photos of defensive formations on the sidelines. They weren't blurry to me, but it was harder for me to focus on them. Another was that my tongue would go numb.*

*The signs are different for everybody, but they're there. The difference for me is that, thanks to Dr. Wolff, I made myself stop every time and identify how I felt different, and recognized that it meant my blood sugar was dropping. This was a tool I used throughout my athletic life.*

*The second thing Dr. Wolff taught me was to make sure I always, always, always had some emergency food around. It sounds simple, but when I was in high school, they didn't have Gatorade on the sidelines. Heck, it was hard to find water. So I always made sure I had a six-pack of some kind of soda. I discussed it with every one of my teachers, and gave each one a pack of Lifesavers to keep in their desk. They were new to this game, too, but as long as*

*I didn't abuse their trust, I could walk up to their desk and*
*get a Lifesaver whenever my body was telling me that my*
*blood sugar was dropping.*

*In the mid- to late-'80s, nutrition was not something*
*that was talked about athletically. But the diet I was on in*
*the '80s for my diabetes – the one built around exchanges as*
*I learned them when I was first diagnosed – is the diet that*
*every elite athlete in the '90s, when I was playing in the*
*NFL, said was the optimal diet for athletic achievement.*

*So I had already starting eating right and being aware*
*of nutrition, being aware of my body, before knowing the*
*NFL was to come. But all these things have helped me*
*because it's so minute, the differences between guys who*
*make it in the NFL and the guys who don't.*

IT IS NO surprise to Dr. Wolff that Jay became a unanimous All-
America football player in college and enjoyed a long and highly
successful professional career.

"Knowledge is power. Being powerful in your life is one of
the most important ingredients in mental health and happiness.
There's almost nothing worse than being powerless.

"What really bums people out with diabetes is the disease,
like, owns them. They're owned by the disease, and they can't
get past it. It takes a fair amount of effort to get to the other side
of it. Unlike Jay, they don't have enough optimism that they can
do that. They don't believe enough. Too many people never get
that far.

"Jay was much smarter, and a much better athlete, and mentally tougher than most people. I remember he called me while he was with the Chicago Bears, and he said, 'You know, no one in the NFL knows as much about diabetes as I do. They have doctors, but they don't know anything.'

"It sounds pretty egotistical, but you know, it was true.

"One time I had this great new book about carbohydrates and exercise. It was published by the American Diabetes Association. It was for physicians, but I sent it to Jay because I knew he'd get it. Jay was basically a diabet-ologist."

Although Dr. Wolff quickly recognized Jay as an exception in the way he quickly understood his disease and accepted responsibility for managing it, she still could never have imagined just how much in control Jay would be, or just how far he would take it.

"I remember he called one time, and told me he was going to a pie-eating contest. He said, 'I don't want your permission, I just want to know how to do it.'

"I could hear his mom in the background. 'Jay, you can't do this. Jay, what's wrong with you!?'

"I said, 'What kind of pies will you be eating, and how many pies do you think you have to eat to win?' I think he called around 4:30, and the contest was something like 6 o'clock.

"I said, 'Here's the first thing you have to do. You can't eat supper.' He asked, 'How should I do my insulin?' We discussed how to do his insulin without getting sick. And we talked everything through.

"I think he won."

*I was a sophomore, and looking back on it, I wanted to be one of the guys. Nobody had to know that I couldn't eat dinner, and had to take insulin, and had to take blood sugars for three hours afterward. I wanted to be normal. And as in everything, if you're going to do it, you might as well win it.*

*I called Dr. Wolff at her home only about four times all the way through high school. It had to be something significant to bother her at home, and this was significant.*

*I had mentioned the pie-eating contest as I went out the door, in a way that I didn't want to have a discussion with my mom. And she didn't want to have a discussion, either, meaning she didn't want to even consider it. So I called Dr. Wolff. I figured if I could tell mom that she said it was okay, before mom could get on the phone with her, I'd be able to do it.*

*I expected it to be that easy, but it got more difficult when Dr. Wolff started asking me questions and I didn't know the answers. 'How big are the pies? What was in the pies? How many calories? How many pies did I have to eat?' I told her I thought it was who could eat one pie the fastest. At least I was hoping that's what it was.*

*I think the biggest sacrifice I had to make was I couldn't eat dinner before the contest. I remember Dr. Wolff saying, 'If you're going to have 5,000 calories in a pie, you don't need to eat dinner.'*

*My mom wasn't thrilled, but Dr. Wolff eventually talked to her, and she accepted that I was going to do it. I think Dr. Wolff said something like, 'You know, Jann. It's not going to kill him. If you let him do it this one time, you won't have*

*to deal with it again. But if you don't let him do it, he'll keep*
*wanting to do it, and you'll keep going through this.'*

*When I got to the contest, I couldn't believe it. They*
*must have opened about four cans of cherries in syrup, and*
*covered them with whipped cream. I don't think it had a*
*crust. But I ate it, and I won. I remember being hungry*
*after I ate the pie.*

THE TRUTH is, Jay was no different than a lot of other teenagers when it came to learning the hard way as he grew up. A self-described "arrogant little smart aleck" who "tended to test the limits," he fought with his big brother, mouthed off to his mother, and experimented with underage drinking.

"We competed in everything," is the way his brother puts it, "even doing the dishes. We had fights over who would do what. We became better friends after high school when we stopped competing every day."

Recalling that sibling rivalry after he married and his first-born was a son, Chris says he convinced his wife they should space a second child farther apart than he and Jay were. He thought that might reduce the potential for warfare if the next baby also was a boy (which it was).

As evidence that "Jay's not perfect," his dad recalls a particularly contentious night at the dinner table. As usual, a spirited discussion was in progress. Jay figures he was a freshman at the time.

"Jay's going through one of these teenage things," Dick

recounts, "and I remember sitting there at the dinner table and Jay just being a smart aleck. He and his mom were going at it, and he called Jann a bitch.

"Like one second after he said it, I smacked him a good one across his face. I don't think I even said anything. We didn't practice corporal punishment in our house, but that was just outside the realm of what you tolerate."

Dick says it got both boys' attention. So much so that Jay can still feel the whack.

*I can replay it in my mind. I didn't have the 'bi'. . . out of my mouth before I was smacked. No question, I had it coming.*

*I'm sure my mom was nailing me on something about either school or responsibility, and I'm sure I was trying to defend myself. My mom and I are similar, and we would go at each other.*

*She was trying to make a point that I thought was just stupid. I was a teenager. And I couldn't make my mom understand. I was getting more and more frustrated.*

*I was getting really worked up.*

*I'm sure my dad was sitting there going, 'Hmm, he's getting more agitated. He isn't letting up. Let's see where this goes. He probably saw it coming and thought,*

*is this idiot really going to go down this road?*

*I got very worked up, and so frustrated and so pissed at my mom that, the next thing you know, she's just a stupid bi . . . and WHAP!*

   *My dad very, very rarely used corporal punishment.*

*But he rocked me. He's got two big hands. It hurt like hell.*

*I never called my mom a bitch again.*


JAY'S MOM and dad tell the story of his first raid on the wine cabinet better than he.

"Jay was playing in a church softball league," Jann recalls. "Dick and I watched his game, then we went out with friends for some ice cream. Jay and some of his friends rode their bikes to our house.

"The next morning, after Jay was usually up, he was still in bed. He wasn't feeling well. We thought he had the flu. Later we got this phone call from the mother of one of his friends.

"The first thing she said was, 'You should know, Jann, that the boys got into some wine at your house last night, and Jay got pretty drunk. I just thought you should know, because he could have hurt himself.' "

Jann later found two empty wine bottles in his bedroom, buried under his dirty clothes.

"That's not very clever," Dick adds, picking up the story.

"We were working in the yard, and we said, 'We can't let him get away with this.' So we decided to put him to work."


*Dad always had a huge vegetable garden. He had just gotten a load of manure. He got me up, took me outside and handed me a pitchfork. He came out of the house about an hour later with a can of beer, and started sipping it. Then he looked at me and said, "You want some?"*

*It's definitely not something I was proud of.*

*When I speak to kids with diabetes now, I don't tell them that story or the pie story. But I do deliver the message that I think is in the pie story. It's basically, 'If you're going to do something dumb – and entering that pie-eating contest was against everything a diabetic should sensibly do – don't do something dumb and be stupid, too.*

*I took the precautions to make sure I didn't wind up in the hospital. I didn't go into this blindly. I made sure I knew the possible outcomes, and how to avoid doing harm to myself.*

*I don't condone underage drinking, for example. I don't think it's right at all. But I know some kids will do it. So I tell them, 'If you choose to do it, you have to do some things. You have to eat. If you drink too much alcohol, your body stops breaking down sugar and spends all its time breaking down the alcohol. But the insulin keeps working, and you wind up with low blood sugar.*

*'A symptom of low blood sugar is that you look like you're drunk. You have to eat and you have to take blood sugars. Bottom line: If you choose to drink, make sure you wake up the next morning.'*

*As a juvenile diabetic, you're forced to learn those life lessons and come to grips with them sooner. 'Is this going to put me in a coma?' That's the reality of a diabetic's life.*

CHAPTER 3

# CHILDREN'S HOSPITAL

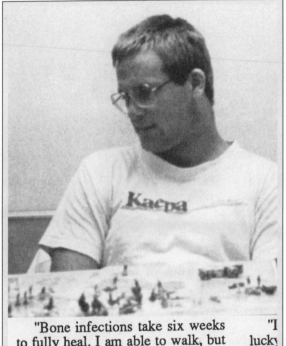

"Bone infections take six weeks to fully heal. I am able to walk, but running and football activity could make the infection come back and be...

"I lucky didn' to b

*Kirkwood Call, reproduced with permission*

*"If this doesn't get better, and get better pretty quick," doctors treating Jay's infected foot told him, "you better get prepared to not have an athletic career."*

In suburban St. Louis, the high schools of neighboring Kirkwood and Webster Groves started playing the Turkey Day football game on Thanksgiving Day in 1903. It's the longest-running game west of the Mississippi, and like most storied rivalries, generations of families with roots on opposite sides of the field would never think of sitting together at noon on that uniquely American day when they later join hands and give thanks for their many blessings, including each other.

Grandfathers played against each other 50-60 years before; their sons 25 years later; and their grandsons 20 years after that. And they still remember the big plays of their youth, those moments when bragging rights were decided for at least the next 12 months, and often for lifetimes.

Turkey Day highlights even made national television one year during halftime of the Dallas Cowboys' annual holiday game. The renewal of the rivalry has been covered in *USA Today*, too.

At Kirkwood High Turkey Day was the culmination of a shortened week of stunts, pranks and traditions aimed at building school spirit to a fervor pitch.

Every class and club decorated the halls of the school with elaborate painted cardboard and papier mache scenes; those judged best received awards. In Jay's senior year, he and his classmates greeted arriving students and teachers from lawn chairs they had sneaked onto the roof of the school. There was a one-hour pep rally every day, and a bonfire the night before the game. At the end of the week, players awoke to banners draped over the front doorways of their homes by the cheerleaders.

That pie-eating contest Jay won as a sophomore was part of the festivities, as well.

It is a scene from the 1987 Turkey Day game, Jay's last as a high school football player, that Coach Dale Collier – DC to his more than three decades of players – recalls as the signature moment in the career of "the best football player I ever coached." The same play also stands out as a moment of realization for Jay's brother Chris.

Webster Groves seemed a sure winner that November day until Kirkwood intercepted a pass late in the game and drove inside the five-yard line as time was running out. On fourth down at the three, DC called time out and went onto the field to huddle with his team.

"What do you want to do?" he asked. "We can kick a field goal and go to overtime."

His star lineman looked him in the eye and said with typical resolve, "Give it to Taylor and run it right up my butt, and we'll score."

Clever Taylor had carried the ball only a couple of times the whole game, as DC recalls, but DC went with the play anyway. Clever followed Jay's block into the end zone, and Kirkwood won, 19-16.

"It was typical of Jay," DC says, the memory of the last play of Jay's high school career still vivid two decades later. "I can't explain it. Every once in a while, as a coach you get one of those kids who just gets the job done, no matter what. That was Jay. He's the toughest, most determined individual I've ever met."

Chris, who was Kirkwood's captain when Jay was moved up to varsity as a sophomore, says it was during Jay's last Turkey Day game that he realized his brother was a special football player.

"I was in my second year at Purdue," Chris begins, "and I was home for Thanksgiving break so, of course, I'm at the game. I sat with a guy named Dave Yarborough, who was an assistant coach at Kirkwood when I played. He actually left Kirkwood after my junior year to become a head coach at another school, Parkway South. We played them my senior year.

"I'm talking with Dave, and he tells me Jay was the only guy they played all year, and the first guy ever in his coaching career, that they game-planned around because he made that much of a difference in the game. They actually tried to avoid him.

"I hadn't heard that about many individuals, and we never did that for any opposing player when I played. That's when I knew my brother was pretty good."

DALE COLLIER coached at Kirkwood and nearby Ladue high schools for a combined 32 years. His Kirkwood teams won 102 games and lost 64 during his 15 years as head coach, and he was named 1986 *Sporting News* Coach of the Year in St. Louis. Between 1964 and 1993 he coached somewhere between eight hundred and a thousand young football players. Dozens went on to play in college, and a few made it to the NFL. But none of them compared to Jay.

"He wasn't the best athlete I ever coached, but he was the best football player. He was a kid who did everything to the utmost, whether it was in the classroom, on the field of play, or just horsing around.

"He's very, very bright. He was a good student. He was very active with everything going on in school. And he truly loved the game; he loved playing football."

Entering Kirkwood High in 1982, Jay had yet to play a down of organized football. It was his father's house rule: no football before high school.

"I would call it active discouraging," Dick Leeuwenburg says. "As much as I love football and love having him play football, I think football is a dumb game for kids. There are lots of other sports that are great for kids.

"I recall a guy I worked with talking about his son in this little league football – every team named for a pro team, and they were all wrapped up in playoffs and a championship game – and thinking, 'What a terrible environment to put a little boy in.' "

*In eighth grade I was the statistician for my brother's sophomore football team. I got to take the bus with the team, and got to see what it was like. I couldn't wait.*

*Dad didn't start playing football until high school, so we didn't either. 'It was good enough for me,' he'd say. 'If you're an athlete, ninth grade is soon enough for football.' So I just accepted it. Ninth grade was good enough for me.*

*I played middle linebacker and center on the freshman team, and I knew from Day One that I loved this sport. I got to hit someone as hard as I could, and got rewarded for it! I craved the collisions. It was truly euphoric. I could never get enough of it. I loved practice. I loved playing.*

*In high school, I never left the field. I played every snap of every game. I played defensive tackle and offensive guard. I snapped on punts and kicks, and I kicked off. I loved kicking off. You know, the kicker is never blocked. I was 230, and in high school, most kids running back kicks are150. I loved creaming them.*

*From the beginning, I wanted to manage my diabetes so that it was never an issue. But not every coach I played for knew how practices would go. Some would stay on schedule, and some were pretty unpredictable.*

*You use practices to simulate a game; I used practices to simulate how I would control my diabetes so that I was successful as a player. Football is such a macho sport; it's hard to say, "Uh, coach, I'm going to take a play off because I need a Coke." The coach is likely to say, "Oh, sure. And would you like a lawn chair, too?"*

*DC taught health, so that helped. I explained to him*
*that I have diabetes. I told him I'd have a six-pack of Cokes*
*on the sidelines. I told him I'd run to the sidelines and chug*
*a Coke if I'm feeling like I'm having low blood sugar. But I*
*didn't want to come out, not out of a game or out of a prac-*
*tice. I wanted to be the best player I could be.*

DICK LIKES to say he had a real good seat for the games when he
is asked about his own pro career. He was part of the 1964
Chicago Bears rookie class that included Gale Sayers, Dick
Butkus and Brian Piccolo, whose death from a rare form of
cancer became the basis for the movie, "Brian's Song."

It didn't make the script, but Dick has his own locker room
memory of Piccolo. It came during what might be termed the
rutting season for rookie football players hoping to show they
belong.

"In the locker room, you're trying to mark your territory,"
Dick begins, "and Piccolo starts making fun of me going to
Stanford. And I answered something about him going to Wake
Forest and everybody majoring in tobacco-chewing and things
like that.

"I was better at it, and I won. I had put him down. The
next day Bill George, the veteran linebacker who had also gone
to Wake Forest, was in my face because Piccolo had told him all
the things I had said about Wake Forest. "

Dick was cut before the last exhibition game. He had
already been accepted into the Stanford Business School, and

Jann had lined up a teaching job, so they went back to California. He thought football was behind him.

"We were unpacking in this little apartment we had rented, and the apartment manager came running up to us and said, 'GEORGE HALAS is on the phone, and he wants to talk to YOU!' Actually it was some assistant coach making the call for Coach Halas. One of their tackles had torn up his knee in the last exhibition game, and they wanted me to come back.

"I had been accepted into the University of Chicago's business program, too, and you could enroll there at any time. So I started in January, after the season."

During the next summer's training camp Dick was traded to the Pittsburgh Steelers, where he roomed with the diabetic lineman who kept his insulin cool on the room air conditioner. He was cut a few weeks later and decided, on the spot, that it really was time to get on with his business career. After graduate school, he began as an economist with Continental Oil in New York. He held executive positions with Boise Cascade for 20 years, then became CEO of Vans Shoes in California until he retired.

As Chris and Jay entered high school, Dick was anything but the classic example of an unfulfilled father who relives his youth through his sons.

"It was never particularly important to either me or Jann that either of our sons be good athletes," he says. "That was never a goal we had as parents, to have one or both of our kids even necessarily play, let alone be very good at it. It was more a thing that Jay decided on his own. That's what he wanted to do. It became important to us only in the sense that it was important to him.

"Jann had Jay take piano lessons for several years. If he had decided that instead of sports it was music that . . . well, had his talents been different, let's put it that way . . . and he had tried to excel in that, we would have supported it and felt just as good about that as sports. We didn't spend a lot of time thinking about how good he was or wasn't, as opposed to if he was feeling good and enjoying it."

Still, Dick had played enough football to realize that Jay was much more than your typical high school player

"As soon as he started playing football, you could look around and tell he was above average; you knew he was good. The coaches were telling us, he's a pretty special football player.

"When he was a sophomore they wanted to put him on the varsity, and I was opposed to it. He was supposed to have fun, and on the sophomore team he could play all the time. But it was what he wanted to do, so at some point you back off and let it be his decision.

When he was a junior, you saw that college football was a realistic possibility for him. I had played a lot of football, and he was playing positions that I had played, so I knew. I thought, 'Wow. He deserves being there. He's pretty good.' "

*The story of my football life is that I continually set short-term goals. I never said, in high school, my goal is to make it to college on a scholarship. And when I was in college, it wasn't, 'I'm gonna do this only because I want to be a pro.'*

*After my junior year in high school, I had made first-team all-conference and honorable mention all-state, and my short-term goal was to be the best football player in the state of Missouri. The next logical progression was to be the best lineman in the state. It wasn't something I advertised to anyone else, just something I had in my mind that I thought realistic and achievable if I kept working hard.*

*We started off 2-0 my senior year; things were going great. Our next game was against a fairly difficult team in our league, Lafayette. It was going to be our first good test, and I couldn't wait to play them.*

*But I wound up in the hospital when I developed a serious case of athlete's foot. I was taking showers in the gym, and I guess I picked up bacteria off the shower floor.*

*When I get athlete's foot, I get a crack in my skin. It's an open sore. I didn't think anything of it; didn't say anything; didn't do anything. I continued to jog, lift weights – all the things you do to be a good football player. And it kept getting worse.*

*After a while, I had to lace my shoe looser to get it on because my foot had swollen so much that I couldn't get my shoe on. I remember my foot was really hurting – throbbing, pounding. But I never missed any football. I just sucked it up. It was the first time in my life that I was noticing pain when I wasn't playing football.*

*I could have told someone about my foot sooner than I did. I should have. Even though I had had diabetes for several years by then, it just never occurred to me that I* needed to take special precautions. Obvious things like wearing flip-flops in the shower or treating my athlete's foot.

I was very good about monitoring my diabetes, taking my blood sugar and watching what I ate. I didn't think I had to worry about taking extra precautions or extra care because I was in control of my diabetes.

One night I was out walking our dog with my mom, and we were just talking, some small talk. And I asked her, "Mom, if you have a really hurt foot and it gets infected, do you think you could, uh . . . You don't really need your pinky toe that much, do you?"

"What?" she said.

I said, "Well, I know you push off with your big toe. You don't really need your pinky toe, do you?"

She looks at me and still doesn't know if I'm joking or what the heck I'm talking about.

I said, "My toe has really been hurting me, and I think the best solution right now, so I don't have to miss any football, is if I can just cut my little pinky toe off, then everything would be fine." That was my solution in my mind.

We get home and we take my shoe and sock off. This is the first time she ever had seen or heard about this injury, which I didn't even consider an injury because it didn't happen while I was playing a sport, and there was no one episode. My foot is swollen, and red, and it's discolored. Now that I look at it, I realize there are some major issues going on.

*The first thing we do, is my mom takes me to the hospital, and they start putting me on oral antibiotics. We talk to Dr. Wolff about the treatment, and, as becomes a pattern in my life, people don't know how to differentiate between either you're a diabetic or you're an athlete, "because we've never had a diabetic athlete."*

*I was not as quick on the uptake then, but one of the very first things they said is, "We really should put you on this medication; oh, but wait, we're not supposed to give this to diabetics. They don't give me any information. What ends up happening is, I'm on the oral medication for a week, and my foot gets progressively much worse. It doesn't improve at all.*

*At that point, they did an extensive number of tests. One test I remember was a bone scan. They wanted to see if the infection had gotten into my bone. That was their worst fear, because if infection gets into you bone, it literally starts eating your bone away. In diabetics that are not in control, those nasty little organisms live on sugar. It's much harder to get the infection killed if your blood sugars are elevated and you give the bacteria extra food.*

*At this point there was no doubt there was something wrong. You can see the foot on the monitor screen while they're doing the scan. I'm talking to the technician, asking him questions. "What don't you want to see," I asked. He said, "You don't want to see red spots. If you see red spots, that means there's infection in there."*

*The guy is doing the scan, and all of a sudden I saw*

what I didn't want to see. It was like this red supernova star right there in my foot. I started to say something, and just that quick, that technician is saying, "I'm not qualified to read this. You really need to talk to a doctor." We both knew.

Part of the way I coped with it was the way I approached it with my mom when we were taking that walk. You know, 'How important is a foot?' The doctors told me, "You need to be prepared. If this doesn't get better, and get better pretty quick, you better get prepared to not have an athletic career."

That was my first real episode of being really mad at this misperception, and/or fact, that people instantly thought the worst because I had diabetes. In my mind, the conversation with the doctors went like this, "Because you're a diabetic and because you don't take care of yourself, this problem's much worse."

My attitude was, 'I've only been a diabetic for FOUR YEARS! How can you say I have long-term complications and circulation issues when I've only had this disease for four years?' So I was an angry man.

At that point in my life, one of the hardest things for me to do was to call up my coach, and I was in tears, explaining to him that I wouldn't be able to play in the game against this big team, that I had to miss this important game.

IT WAS never a major concern to DC that he was coaching a player with diabetes. He didn't limit Jay's participation, and didn't treat him any differently than any other player.

"In those days we didn't know that much about juvenile diabetes. Jay controlled it very well, and never wanted it to be something that stood out. So it didn't. To his teammates, he was just that goofy guy playing football."

The shock that DC and his players felt then, when Jay called from the hospital to tell his coach he wouldn't be able to play against Lafayette, is understandable.

"He calls and tells me, 'DC, I can't play. I'm sick.' It was very scary. We'd just come off a big win. We had a good season going. And all of a sudden Jay went from being this horse for us to almost losing his foot. To see someone so big and strong get knocked down so fast was scary, very scary.

"Typical of Jay, though, all he wanted to talk about was how upset he was that he was going to miss this big game, and how sorry he was that he was letting the team down. It was unbelievable. Football is a game to me. It's great, but it's still a game. I said, 'Son, I can't believe you're worried about that when you might lose your foot. You've got to be worried about your foot.'"

Playing without their leader, the Kirkwood Pioneers had to score 10 points in the fourth quarter for a come-from-behind win against Lafayette. They won the next week, then lost two in a row to teams DC is convinced they would have beaten if Jay had been playing. By the time Jay returned, Kirkwood was on the verge of missing the state playoffs.

All that remained of the schedule were games against Fox and Mehlville. Kirkwood had to win them both. "Jay missed five games," DC says with lasting urgency. "If we hadn't gotten into the playoffs, there wouldn't have been a season for him."

*I spent two weeks in the hospital on intravenous antibiotics because they were the strongest. Because I was still in high school, I was in the children's ward. Other than a girl down the hall who had cancer, there weren't any kids older than eight on the whole floor. She was an eighth-grader.*

*I was really uncomfortable about being there. I wanted to be treated like an adult. Besides wanting it to be over, I didn't want to go through this and feel like I was being treated like a kid. I was bored out of my mind. I had done my homework – when you have nothing else to do, it doesn't take more than an hour – and I didn't have anything else interesting to do. I was going stir crazy.*

*I guess I saw her in the hall. We started talking in a community room where you could watch TV. She had been there a heck of a lot longer than I had, and probably several times before. I would ask her honest questions, like, "Are you going to die?" No one would ever talk to her like that. Everyone would avoid her.*

*A doctor once told me that she said I was one of the only people she felt comfortable with not putting her wig on. She had lost her hair. It was helpful, for both of us, I think, just to have somebody to talk to who wasn't six years old.*

*I don't remember her name. I wish I did. One day I wasn't feeling good, and she knew I was having a bad day. She came down to see me, and gave me one of those little friendship bracelets. It was one of those braided ropes, something she had made herself. It had obviously taken her some time.*

*She was seemingly doing fine. Two days later I heard that she died. I realized right then there was no reason for me ever to feel sorry for myself.*

*When I got out of the hospital, I still had to have four intravenous treatments a day so it was hard to go to school. But I had to be there for physics and AP calculus. Those were the two classes I couldn't handle from home. The one rule in our house was, you had to get an education. If you didn't keep a 3.0 average, at least a B, you didn't play football.*

*So I went to school with the IV hookup in my hand. They had to keep moving it because the medication was so strong it was eating my veins. My arm was full of holes. It was very painful.*

*The problem finally cleared up after a month. I had a clean bill of health, with one exception. The doctors felt the bone had been weakened by the infection, and they were afraid I might break my foot. But I wasn't going to let that stop me from playing again.*

*Fox had a big defensive lineman named Mike Wells. He wound up playing a short time in the NFL, too, with the Lions. I hadn't done anything for a month, but I thought everything would be the same. We ran a trap play, and my*

*job was to block the end. It was the only time in my high*
*school career that I got my clock cleaned. Wells just flat-*
*tened me.*


DALE COLLIER half laughs and half marvels as he recalls Jay's
return and his humbling encounter with Mike Wells.

"Once they found out he wasn't going to lose his foot, and
then that he wasn't going to lose some toes, Jay was back on the
field. He couldn't practice, but he sat there and watched every
practice and kept up with what he was supposed to do on every
play. Jay is so smart; he didn't forget anything.

"As soon as he got clearance to play, he thought he'd be
okay. He thought it would be just like the day after he played
his last game, because he was keeping up with everything. But
I don't think Jay weighed more than 205 by the end of the
season. He had lost about 25 pounds. He needed to ease back
into the game, but of course he never 'eased' into anything."

The Missouri high school football playoff system was as
much a test of teams' conditioning and stamina as it is a measure of football supremacy. The first round was played on the
Wednesday following the weekend on which the regular season
ends, and the second round was three days after that. Kirkwood
beat Fox and Mike Wells, even though Jay played only a small
part of the game, then crushed Mehlville, with Jay back full time.
DC's squad had made the playoffs.

"We beat Mehlville back-to-back, on Friday and again the
next Wednesday. Then we played Hazlewood Central on

Saturday. Jay played the most awesome game I've ever seen
played. I'm an old lineman, and I know what it's like to go up
against a guy who's a whole lot bigger and stronger. For Jay to
play the game he played, against the guy he was up against, was
truly amazing, considering what he had been through. He just
had so much heart."

*Kirkwood was the smallest of the large division
schools in Missouri, and Hazlewood Central was the largest
school in the big school division. They had an offensive
lineman named Russo, and the day before we played, the St.
Louis Post Dispatch announced that Russo had been named
lineman of the year in the state. The one goal I had set, to
be the best lineman in the state, had been awarded to a guy
on the other team.*

*Central had another stud named Mario Johnson, who
wound up playing a few years in the NFL. I lined up
against him when he was with the Jets. We scrimmaged
when he was with the Saints.*

*Mario was about 6 feet 2 and 280 in high school. He
played fullback and defensive tackle, so I would be blocking
him when he played tackle, and I'd be tackling him when he
played fullback.*

*I had a great game against Mario on offense, and
when I was on defense I got to go up against the best lineman in the state, and did really well. I tackled Mario two
or three times in the backfield.*

I felt good that I had made it back, that I had been able to return and play my best after what I had been through. But we lost 21-14. We had a bomb that would have tied the game. It hit our receiver in the hands but he dropped it.

I was looking forward to playing in Arrowhead Stadium, where the Chiefs play. But that wasn't going to happen. My last high school game was going to be Turkey Day against Webster Groves.

# CHAPTER 4

# THE FLEETING IRISH

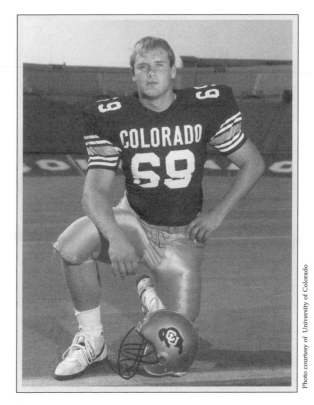

Photo courtesy of University of Colorado

*"I looked at it as sort of . . . a GOOD thing,"*
*Gary Barnett, who recruited Jay for Colorado,*
*says of Jay's hospitalization. "Because I figured*
*everybody would back off."*

*"Cheer, cheer for old Notre Dame,*
*Wake up the echoes calling her name . . ."*

— Notre Dame Victory March, 1908

LETTERS FROM college recruiters began arriving at the Leeuwenburg's Kirkwood home at the beginning of Jay's senior season. He was most excited about the ones coming from South Bend, Indiana.

A few universities have played intercollegiate football longer than the Fighting Irish. But none can match the legend and lore of Rockne, Grantland Rice's Four Horsemen and "Win One for The Gipper," or the contemporary symbolism of The Golden Dome and Touchdown Jesus.

And no other school's exploits have been chronicled in the

same, storied way. In slightly more than 100 years of football, more than 100 books have been written about Notre Dame football, its coaches, heroes and history. At least a dozen movies feature the Fighting Irish or their gridiron immortals.

In a century of sports writing, "Outlined against a blue, gray October sky the Four Horsemen rode again," remains the single most memorable line ever written about a college football team or group of players.

The Irish are the Yankees of college football – hated by legions weary of the mystique, yet the dream team for so many who play their trademark sport.

*One school I always wanted at least to visit and decide if I wanted to go there was Notre Dame. Every other year, it seemed, they were playing for the national championship. I remember my dad saying when he played at Stanford, they played Notre Dame every year and never beat them. They were a power.*

*I didn't have any connections there. I didn't know anybody who went there. I wasn't Catholic. But I wanted to go there because it was the big-time school with the biggest reputation. And it had a great academic background.*

*Right before I went into the hospital for my foot problem, I was getting their letters, one a week. I was just about ready to say I wanted to make an official visit. That means they pay for you to fly out there; they pay for your hotel, your meals. Everything's taken care of.*

*I was about to tell them I wanted to set up an official*
*visit, then I went in the hospital and they stopped recruit-*
*ing me. I never received another letter from them – nothing*
*more, at any stage.*

*Lou Holtz was in his first year as head coach at Notre*
*Dame. He has denied he even knew they were recruiting me*
*and stopped because of my foot. But I didn't think it was a*
*coincidence then, and I still don't.*

*I was more resentful of Notre Dame, which started*
*courting me then backed off all of a sudden like that, than*
*say, an Oklahoma, which said, "we have bigger fish that*
*we're going to go after." I respected that.*

*It really ticked me off because it felt like Notre Dame*
*was taking any of the decision making out of my hands*
*because of my diabetes. That experience definitely came*
*back later in my life. I wanted a chance to prove a school*
*wrong, one that I really wanted to go to. I got that chance,*
*in back-to-back Orange Bowls.*

LETTER WRITING is the way all college programs begin the
courtship of virtually every high school athlete. On a major
college coaching staff, each assistant is assigned a region of the
country to recruit. Personal contact and actual conversation
between a college coach and a high school prospect are severely
limited by National Collegiate Athletic Association rules, so
coaches become pen pals.

"I tried to send a letter every week to every kid I was

recruiting," says Gary Barnett, who was an assistant on Bill McCartney's staff at Colorado in 1986. "If I was on vacation in Hawaii, I'd get a bunch of surfboard postcards and send one a day while I was gone. I'd write, 'That's me on the number 2 surfboard,' and stuff like that. It was all about building relationships with the kids."

Barnett became a major college head coach in 1992, and was voted national Coach of the Year in 1995 after leading Northwestern University, long the doormat of college football, to the Big Ten Conference championship and a berth in the Rose Bowl. It was Northwestern's first bowl appearance in almost a half century.

His team won a share of the Big Ten title and played in another bowl game again the next year, then Colorado hired him back as its head coach in 1999. In Barnett's third season CU won the Big 12 Conference championship.

In 1986, though, he was in only the third year of his first job as a major college assistant coach. He had grown up in St. Louis, and knew the high school programs of the area. He'd even attended Turkey Day games.

"St. Louis was my area to recruit," he says. "It was important to me to go recruit players out of that area because that's where I was from. It was my home, and I needed to prove to Coach McCartney that I could sign players from there and get them to come to the University of Colorado. I knew most of the coaches there. I had played there. So I had a relationship with most of them."

One of those relationships was with Dale Collier at

Kirkwood High.

"Every year I went through St. Louis, I stopped at Kirkwood. We already had a Kirkwood player at Colorado, Michael Simmons. I had recruited Michael, and had gotten close to Dale. So when I started recruiting Jay, I went a lot on what Dale Collier told me. I trusted Dale a lot. If Dale said he was a football player, then he was a football player; he was a Division One football player.

"So I had made up my mind in May that I was going to recruit Jay Leeuwenburg, just because of all the things Dale told me about him. The words he used were, 'He's a throwback. He's just a throwback to old-time football players.' That means, when you blow the whistle, they're there and ready to play.

"I knew Jay had diabetes at that point in time, and I brought it up in all our recruitment meetings. There were questions as to whether or not we should continue to recruit Jay. But our trainer said there were guys playing with diabetes in the NFL, and he said the biggest problem, as I recall, is getting your diet under control. We didn't think that would be an issue."

Barnett reacted to the news about Jay's hospitalization and the problem with his foot very differently than Notre Dame apparently did.

"I looked at it as," Barnett says, pausing to search for the right description, "as sort of . . . a GOOD thing. Because I figured everybody would back off.

"At the time, you could make one phone call a week to any high school player you were recruiting. So I saw this as an opportunity. I called him in the hospital. I called him every week. We never faltered."

Barnett never actually saw Jay play football. He's not even sure he watched film of Jay playing football. "It wouldn't have made any difference," he shrugs, "because I was going to see what I wanted to see. I had made my mind up. I was going to recruit Jay Leeuwenburg."

Barnett's first-hand scouting consisted of sitting in the stands at several of Kirkwood High's wrestling matches after football season ended. After playing on the basketball team since he was a freshman, Jay decided to try one more sport before he graduated.

"If you don't know the player very well or you have question marks about him," Barnett explains, "you want to see his competitiveness, see his body, see how he moves. And wrestling is a great sport for seeing all those things. It's better than any other sport.

"The other reason is you already know you want him, so you just need to have a presence. You want him to feel you're really interested in him. Between December and February I went to St. Louis every week for 10 to 12 weeks, mainly to show Jay I really wanted him to come to Colorado."

*I knew Gary was there at some of the matches, but I knew he wasn't supposed to talk to me face-to-face. There was maybe a wave, 'Hey, I'm here,' and that was it.*

*There were two very significant reasons that I decided to try wrestling.*

*One, I stunk at basketball. Maybe not stunk, but I had bulked up enough and I very much liked the physical nature of football. I was not a finesse guy.*

*My junior year, I vividly remember a time when a team set a double pick on me, and I just ran over the two guys like I was a defensive tackle. I remember the whistle blowing, and I went, 'Yeh, those guys fell and they tripped me.'*

*I got a foul, and I thought, 'You know, I really don't think this is my sport.' Because my instant reaction was, 'Plow over these guys.'*

*The second reason I wrestled was, every one of my close friends wrestled. A friend a year older than I was a two-time state champion at 145 pounds. Another one, my best friend since first grade, who wound up being Best Man in my wedding, wrestled at 138. My third best friend was in there, too.*

*They kept telling me how much fun it was, and how I could hang out with them, and how they really needed a heavyweight. I knew basketball wasn't for me. It sounded like a perfect fit. I wanted to see if I could do it.*

*I made it through the district and sectional, and went to the state tournament. I won two matches and lost two matches. The guys I lost to weighed in at 275 pounds. I weighed 222, almost 55 pounds lighter. They literally just sat on me, and I didn't have enough savvy to do anything about it. I just got smothered. I got squished.*

HIGH SCHOOL football players were allowed to make up to five official campus visits when Jay was a senior. Most visits occurred in December and January, in advance of national letter-of-intent signing day in mid-February, when schools and players formally committed to each other.

Jay hadn't yet scheduled his visit to Boulder and the Colorado campus, and as Barnett continued his weekly visits to Kirkwood, he was worried that Jay would decide to go where a lot of other players from his school had gone.

"Most of the kids from Kirkwood went to Iowa," he recalls. "So I was afraid he was going to go to Iowa. I KNEW he was going to go to Iowa, because the quarterback from his team went to Iowa. Iowa had beaten me on three or four kids in St. Louis.

"Coach Collier had told me during the spring when I started recruiting Jay, 'You're going to have to beat Iowa on him.' So when he wound up in the hospital, in my prayers at night it was, 'Please, let Iowa drop Jay Leeuwenburg.' "

Recruiting a high school football player usually isn't just a matter of convincing him to choose your school. The assistant coach doing the recruiting also has to convince his boss, the head coach, that the kid is worth a scholarship ahead of kids being recruited by other coaches on the staff. And often those other coaches are trying just as hard to sell their own prospects at the expense of each other's. There are, after all, only so many scholarships to be given out.

In Colorado's case in 1987, there were just 12, to be exact, about half the number usually available.

"We were going to be very selective that year," Barnett

recalls. When there were only 12 scholarships, your chances of getting shut out were pretty good. I told myself, I'll be damned if I'm going to get shut out.

"When we met with Coach McCartney to go over the kids we were recruiting, it was like a sales meeting. You had to stand up and sell the player you wanted, because everybody wanted to get a kid. Everybody wanted to recruit at least one player. You didn't want to get shut out.

"To some extent, it came down to ego. It came down to getting a kid. You know that once you get them here, they either make it or they don't. So you just wanted to recruit a quality player. I wanted a kid that I recruited on our team. I wanted to keep the St. Louis thing going."

As a head coach, Barnett watches film on every player he considers for a scholarship. But Bill McCartney wasn't that way.

"There were tricks to selling a kid to Mac," he says with a twinkle in his eyes. "Whoever got their players in earliest for visits had the best shots to get them with Mac," "He didn't know the recruits until we told him about them in our meetings. He didn't go scout them, or watch film on them himself. So the first kids he met were the ones who stood out in his mind.

"And one of the things Mac always did was, he tried to predict every year who the captains were going to be. The players elected them. So I predicted to Mac that Leeuwenburg was going to be a captain. That was one of the things you could always get to Mac with: 'Mac, he's going to be your captain.' So that was part of my sales pitch."

McCartney says he was sold as soon as he visited Jay's

home with Barnett.

"You walked in that home and you immediately sensed the warmth, affection and admiration those parents had for their son, and you could tell his mom and dad were classy people. It was very clear.

"Jay had that sparkle in his eyes and that bounce in his step. You knew that one day he would lead if things went well. He was a flat-out blue chipper – as a person and as an athlete. Talent gives you a chance to be good. But you have to have the chemistry, the intangibles, to make it happen. You could see that Jay had it all."

*My number one criteria coming out of high school was the quality of education I'd receive in college. I had come to the conclusion that I was going to be an engineer.*

*I truly looked up to my father. He was a very successful businessman, a very intelligent man. He didn't tell me where to go, but he made it explicitly clear that he would be severely disappointed if I didn't go to a good school, knowing that the majority of college athletes don't play in the NFL. My number one priority was getting that degree from a good school that would set me up for life.*

*So for that reason, I didn't even consider some of the schools that were recruiting me. I decided I'd make official visits to Stanford, Vanderbilt, Colorado and Iowa.*

*Missouri was real interested in me, and I actually took an unofficial visit there. But their head coach had just* been arrested for his third DUI. The St. Louis Post Dispatch had come to the conclusion that he was not going to continue to be there. That was very unattractive to me.

Also, I felt I had made a name for myself in the state of Missouri, and I had lived in St. Louis my whole life. So I was ready to move on. I was one of the few who wanted to get away from home.

My father had just taken a new job, so he wasn't going to have ties to St. Louis anymore. I knew my mom and dad were moving to California. So it wasn't as if I was going to be able to be close to them by going to Missouri.

Not one school ever brought up my diabetes. They probably discussed it, but they never brought it up with me. I never hid it. Unless they were just totally incompetent, they had to know I had diabetes. And with the injury, they had to know.

My thinking was, from day one, it was something I was going to take care of. And if I need your help, I'll tell you, and I'll tell you what kind of help I need. Right or wrong, I thought it was something I could handle.

Vanderbilt was my first trip, and I was very excited about going there. But the head coach was so uncharismatic, he lost all chance. And the guys who showed me around were too geeky – 'I'm a freshman, but I'm a junior because of all the AP classes I took' – stuff like that.

Stanford was the only Pac 10 school I was interested in. My dad played there, so going in, I thought I wanted to go there, too.

*Jack Elway, John Elway's dad, was the head coach at Stanford when I was being recruited. They actually recruited me as a linebacker. I went in for my meeting with Coach Elway the second day of my visit, and he was talking about his program, and I said, 'I want to come here.'*

*He told me they did not have a scholarship for me at that time. They were not ready to offer me a scholarship. True to my nature, I was very agitated. I asked him, pointblank, 'Then why did you bother flying me out here if you weren't going to offer me a scholarship?' I told him I thought it was dirty pool.*

*He explained that they were prepared to give two scholarships to linebackers, and their number one guy that they really wanted had not committed anywhere yet. So they were not ready to make that decision until he decided.*

*I thought it was very curious that they said they were recruiting me as a linebacker, because even though they said they had two slots for linebackers, I met with the line coach and he told me they were going to make me a lineman. So to me, it seemed that I was a bubble guy.*

*At that point, I was so thoroughly disgusted, it didn't matter. And I told them so.*

*When I met with Coach McCartney at Colorado, the impression I had was no nonsense. This is the way it is. He really came across as genuine. That wasn't the case with the other head coaches.*

*Mac was a great salesman because it felt like he knew me – even though I now know he had no clue.*

*He said, "We have a center. We're looking at you*
*playing in two years. You'll red-shirt, get used to being*
*here at CU, get a good foothold on your studies, get to play*
*against the best teams in the country. And, we're moving*
*up. If you like the way that sounds, we want you here. If*
*you don't, we're wasting your time.'*

*I had not given Coach Mac or Barnett any indication*
*where I was leaning when I left Boulder. But after three*
*visits, I had decided, 'I'm done. I want to go here.'*

*I was at the airport when I called my folks, because my*
*flight was delayed. I told my folks that I was going to CU.*
*That's when Gary knew. He was at the airport with me,*
*and you could still go to the gate then. He heard me, and*
*he called Mac while I was still on the phone with my folks.*

*I told Iowa I was no longer interested in going on an*
*official visit. They wanted to know what they did wrong,*
*what they could have done better. It truly wasn't anything*
*they did or didn't do. They were fourth, and after three*
*visits, I was worn out. I got tired of making visits.*

THE HEADLINE in the *Rocky Mountain News* of February 12, 1987
read: "McCartney calls '87 class his best." The story about
Colorado's recruiting class that year said McCartney called it the
best he had assembled in his five years as head coach, even
though it was his smallest. "This year's class is hand picked," he
was quoted as saying.

That class included six players – half the class – who went

on to play a combined 699 games in the National Football League. The six were Alfred Williams, Eric Bienemy, Mike Pritchard, Joel Steed, Kanavis McGhee and Jay Leeuwenburg.

During the next four seasons, they also formed the nucleus of the best teams in University of Colorado football history. Notre Dame would come to know them well.

CHAPTER 5

# LESSONS

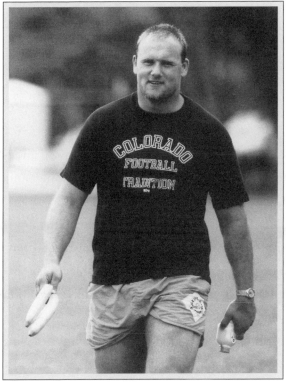

Photo courtesy of The Daily Camera, Boulder

*"It definitely was not always smooth sailing
diabetes-wise," Jay says.  Bananas and orange juice
were more appealing than watered-down
Gatorade and other concoctions.*

THE RECRUITS of 1987 hadn't exactly chosen an established powerhouse when they decided to come to Boulder and play for Bill McCartney.

Colorado football had slipped badly by the time he left the University of Michigan in 1982 for what turned out to be the only major college head coaching job of his career. In the previous three seasons under Chuck Fairbanks, the Buffaloes won only seven and lost 26.

McCartney's declaration to Jay that, "We're moving up," was more an article of faith at that point than a statement of fact. In McCartney's first three seasons, his teams bettered Fairbanks by only a tie (7-25-1), including a 1-10 record in his third year, 1984.

"In Chuck Fairbanks' three years as head coach, and in my first three years as head coach, we were dead last in Division I," McCartney volunteers. "Of a hundred and some-odd colleges, we were last. Fourteen victories in six years."

His fourth team finally produced a winning record – 7-5,

counting a loss in the Freedom Bowl. It was Colorado's first winning season in seven years, and its first post-season bowl appearance in nine. The next year, Jay's senior high school season, Colorado was a .500 team, six wins and six losses. But McCartney knew he had turned the corner in rebuilding the CU program.

"When you want to build a skyscraper," he says, "the higher you want to build, the deeper you have to dig. You have to have a strong foundation. We had started getting kids from in-state who really had a passion for reviving Colorado football."

*I knew the second week of our first training camp that our class was going to be something special. We had had a week when just our recruiting class came in. It was a boot camp to get us up to speed with the playbook, the terminology – everything about CU.*

*We didn't really know that week, because we were just beating on each other. Then they brought in the veterans. By the end of that first week with the full squad there, we knew we were pretty damn good.*

*Bienemy was in the top two at running back right away. Alfred and Kanavis were first or second team, and still didn't quite know all the defensive schemes and all the plays. Pritchard, you could tell he was just an athlete. Then you had me and Joel Steed. We were both red-shirted because they had returning starters in front of us.*

*Bill Coleman, Curt Koch and Don DeLuzio are three guys who really stick out in my mind from my first year in*

*college. They were all from in-state, from the Denver area,
and they were the leaders when we got to CU. They said
from Day One:*

*"You are a special class. You are going to lead us to
greatness. You are going to be better than we could ever
hope to be. We have worked so hard to make this program
come out of the depths of nothing. But we expect you to
take us places we couldn't go without you."*

*It was really empowering, and really genuine.*

SAL AUNESE preceded Jay and his fellow recruits by a year. But
his first playing time was delayed a season because he didn't
have the grades coming out of high school to satisfy the National
Collegiate Athletic Association.

Aunese quarterbacked Vista High of Oceanside to a 13-0
record in 1985, running and passing for more than 2,000 yards
and 20 touchdowns. For that, he was chosen California high
school co-player of the year. A 5-foot-11 left-handed option
quarterback, he was just what McCartney needed to be competitive in the Big 8.

"He had fire in his eyes, a flat-out competitor," McCartney
recalls. "He didn't have great ability, but he was a rugged guy,
hard to tackle. If it was third-and-3, you knew you were going to
move the chains. You knew Sal would find a way. He wanted the
ball. That's the best way to describe him. He wanted the ball."

Having satisfied the NCAA academically, Aunese began
the '87 season as the No. 2 quarterback. But when the starter,

Marc Walters, was injured in the third game of the season, at home against Washington State, Aunese ran for 185 yards as his replacement and rallied the Buffaloes to a 26-17 win. McCartney named him CU's starter two days later.

In nine games that season, Aunese led the team in rushing and passing yardage, and tied Bienemy for most touchdowns. On November 30, 1987 he was named the Big 8 Conference's newcomer of the year.

*We wound up going 7-4 our first year. It was CU's best record in ten years, and we all knew we were going to get better. Eric Norgard, who was first-team All-Big Eight the next year and went on to play in the pros for ten years, was the starting center. He's why I was red-shirted.*

*My red-shirt year didn't go at all the way I expected. Jay's theory of the way red-shirting should work was: You're not going to play. You don't travel to any of the games. You can dress for the home games, but there's no way in hell you're getting in. So, basically, you can take it easy for a year.*

*The reality of the situation was: Jay, you're second-team center. Our No. 1 center gets, hurt, you're not getting red-shirted. You have to go to every meeting, and go all-out every practice. You have to make sure you don't go out and party; you need to make sure you're mentally and physically ready to get in there.*

*I didn't play a single down my freshman year. Missed*

*all the good parties. Didn't get to do anything on any of the weekends. At that point, I was going, "What happened to this big college social life I was going to be a part of?" But having said that, it did help me with my studies. I got a 3.5 my first year. That got me a lifetime exemption from study table.*

*It definitely was not always smooth sailing, diabetes-wise, for me that first year. Red-shirting gave me time to learn some valuable lessons and make some adjustments.*

*I felt it extremely important to push myself as hard as I could in practice to try to simulate a game and simulate the way my diabetes would be, playing at the college level, knowing that I could try to really fine-tune it. What that tended to mean was I would get low more often in practice than I ever would in games.*

*It was during those sessions that I came to realize that colleges do not have unlimited budgets. Yes, they would give the guys Gatorade, but it was watered down. I drank so much Gatorade one time when I was low and couldn't get my sugar up enough that I ended up throwing up every-thing I drank. And I drank like a gallon of it.*

*I was asking myself, "Why is my sugar not coming up?" I knew this was not working for me, but I didn't know why. I didn't realize they dilute the stuff during two-a-days because they knew the guys would just drink it all. It was hydration, not the sugar, for the normal athlete.*

*I had not yet learned enough to know that they have these packets of Gatorade powder that you could mix to make it stronger. Later, I mixed it to a very high concentration.*

Then it became pretty funny to watch other guys run up, grab a bottle with my version in it and take a swig. They were the ones spitting it out then. "Ugh, what is that," they'd say.

For a while they tried giving me this stuff I affectionately called liquid snot. I don't even know the name of this stuff. It was like using Elmer's Glue. It came in a little tube, just like Elmer's Glue. You had this little twisty top.

You squirted it in your mouth, but then you had to wash it down with something. But what ended up happening was, you'd squirt this sticky, gooey yuch in your mouth, and then you'd get a glass of water or even better, a glass of Gatorade, to wash it down. And you'd put the water in your mouth, and all of a sudden it would form a ball. It was like I was drinking this racquetball-sized goo glob. It was horrible.

The trainers were trying to be proactive. "Hey, we got this new product; it's supposed to be great." They're feeling great about themselves. I'm low and they could just stick it in their little fanny packs, and pull it out. "Here, have a squirt of this." You don't have to have somebody run to the sidelines to get a thing of Gatorade.

It sounds great. But, no. I'd rather throw up water than have this stuff. It worked, but I hated it. This stuff was disgusting. Even though it worked, that was secondary. I remember one time talking with a distance runner about it. He hated it, too. Having to take it was almost worse than having low blood sugar. It only lasted about a month. I have never had it since.

STILL BACKING up Norgard, Jay saw his first collegiate game action in 1988, though not quite enough to letter as a red-shirt freshman. With Aunese leading the team in total offense, Colorado won eight and lost three, narrowly losing to both Oklahoma and Nebraska. It was the Buffaloes' best record in 12 years, and it earned them an invitation to the Freedom Bowl in Anaheim, an easy drive from Oceanside for Sal's big sister, Ruta.

No one was happier to see Colorado invited to the Freedom Bowl than Ruta. She had seen every high school game her brother played, but had yet to see him as a college quarterback. Looking forward to the game, neither she nor any of his teammates or coaches could have imagined what this game would come to represent in his still-young life.

On a clear, 47-degree evening two nights before New Year's Eve, Aunese completed just 4 of 13 passes for a mere 46 yards, was sacked four times, and, uncharacteristically, didn't make even 50 yards on 14 rushing attempts. McCartney replaced him in the fourth quarter as Brigham Young went on to win, 20-17. He would never take the field again.

Ruta Aunese would later recall telling her brother, "I'm glad they took you out." She would add, "I'd never seen him so sluggish. Looking back, I think he was sick then."

Late the following March, Aunese was diagnosed with inoperable stomach cancer. Tests showed it had spread to his lungs. Six months later, three games into Colorado's next season, Aunese died at the age of 21.

It remains difficult for McCartney to recount that time. "Sal was sick during spring practice. But when we came back in the fall, that's when the full realization hit me. He was like a skeleton. When his teammates saw him, it took their breath away. They saw the sober reality of what was in front of us."

Immediately after Sal's death, his family was besieged with movie proposals. And in the Hollywood spirit of Notre Dame and The Gipper, his Colorado teammates named him their honorary captain and dedicated their season to him. His locker was enclosed with Plexiglass, his jersey, helmet and cleats displayed within as both a tribute to him and a reminder to his teammates.

*When Sal died, it was the first time I had ever seen an open casket. It was the first funeral I had ever been to. That was life-changing for me. To see this guy who was just a great football player, literally shrivel away to nothing was very humbling and really put things in perspective.*

*I was never a guy who hung out with football players that much. This experience left me with a sense that I better get to know my teammates a little better, that I better not be so selfish with my life. I owed it to everybody to come out of my shell and get to know the members of my team.*

*It was really emotional for everybody. And obviously we ended up, as a team, rallying around it.*

*And that's where Coach McCartney did such a masterful job. He just did such a great job of being able to teach life skills from that moment. The way that he handled it with such grace and such dignity made an impression on everybody who was involved. I was very impressed, and still am, with that whole set of circumstances and how it went about.*

*What helped me is coach McCartney treated us like men. He didn't try to make it a big religious thing, like a test of faith or anything. It was just, 'This is a young man who is extremely sick.' He told us everything he knew, but he didn't have any answers, and he didn't try to pretend that he did.*

*We had a private ceremony before the public memorial service, and it was done in a way that you felt like you were doing the right thing, respecting him and his family and honoring him in the right way.*

ALMOST AS though he looked at the schedule and saw one last way to help his team, Aunese died on Colorado's open date, the only Saturday of that season when CU was off. It allowed Colorado's players to collect themselves from the realization that youthful invincibility is a myth, and to prepare for their first road game, at Washington, the next weekend.

Even though Colorado was ranked fifth nationally and had won its first three games (by convincing margins), some feared that Washington (2-1 and ranked 21st) would be too much for a team in mourning, no matter how talented it was. Especially playing at home. Washington, after all, had won three-fourths of all the games it had played in its home stadium the previous 14 seasons.

"They had tremendous tradition, and great teams under

Don James," McCartney says. "I knew going in this was going to be a hard game to win, even without everything we were dealing with concerning Sal's death."

Wearing Aunese's uniform number on towels hanging from their belts, CU's players gathered on the field before the kickoff, collectively dropped to one knee and bowed their heads in tribute to their honorary captain. And then, in unison, they all raised their index fingers to the sky. It was the defining moment of a bittersweet season.

*The part I remember that impresses me the most about that day, is that it was truly spontaneous.*

*As a team we had agreed: 'We're going to gather and say a prayer before the game, and we're going to be strong about this, and we're going to remember Sal.' Nobody said, 'and then . . .'*

*I don't remember who it was, but when we were in the huddle, someone said, 'We're going to remember you,' and pointed to the heavens. And everybody just joined in."*

*After that, we just ran all over them.*

THE SCORE was 38-6 when McCartney pulled the first-teamers at the start of the fourth quarter. Final score: Colorado 45, Washington 28. Only one opponent in history, Southern California in 1929, had ever scored more points on Washington's home field than Colorado that day.

"That moment stands out unlike any other I've witnessed or heard about," McCartney says. "You can't go into a place like that and beat a team that good in their own back yard that badly without something special having happened. That was a team that was truly one heartbeat.

Over the next two months, the runaway Buffaloes were unbeatable, winning their remaining seven games by an average margin of 29.7 points to complete the only 11-0 season in 99 years of Colorado football. The winning margin would have been somewhere in the 30s but for a narrow, 27-21 victory over Nebraska, proclaimed Colorado's arch rival by McCartney shortly after he arrived on the scene.

*Mac had made Nebraska literally the red-letter game. You couldn't wear red. Anything. He would physically throw you out of a meeting the week of Nebraska if you had anything red on your person. You might have a red fleck in your shirt. You certainly didn't wear that anywhere near the Dal Ward Center that week.*

*I truly believe Mac respected Nebraska and wanted in a lot of ways to emulate them in their dominance over the years. But the way he did it was, "You beat them. If you have one game you're going to win, you beat Nebraska."*

*And truly, you beat Nebraska in those days, you were going to be the Big 8 champion.*

*We were ranked No. 2 in the country, and Nebraska was ranked No. 3 when we played in the 1989 season. I remember very vividly Jeff Campbell having two just monstrous punt returns in that game. Offensively, Nebraska outgained us by 170 yards, but Jeff's punt returns made up for that. He went on to have a great pro career, but it was those two punt returns that made him a folk hero in the state of Colorado.*

*On Jeff's second punt return, he didn't score. He ended up getting to the four-yard line. Which was great, because we had to go out there and punch it in. We're in our own North end zone, the closed end of the field, and we couldn't hear our own plays. It was insane. I couldn't believe how loud Folsom Field could get.*

*I remember thinking that I had been to stadiums that had 30,000 or 40,000 more people in them than we had in Folsom Field that day. But it was the loudest I had ever heard any stadium in my life. I got an instant headache because it was so loud.*

*There was no way I could hear the snap count. The only way I got the snap off was Darian goosed me when he wanted the ball. I was so glad we scored on the first play.*

*Nebraska had beaten CU 20 out of the last 21 games before we beat them that day. But we truly expected to beat them. We were as sure of ourselves as I can imagine any team being. Our attitude was, 'Of course we won.' It never entered our minds that we would lose, because we were going to win the national championship.*

COLORADO STILL had two road games to play after beating
Nebraska. But an emotional letdown was never an issue. The
Buffaloes crushed Oklahoma State 41-17 and Kansas State 59-11.
Their reward for a perfect season was the No. 1 national ranking,
and an opportunity to clinch a national championship in the
muggy air of the Orange Bowl on New Year's Night.

As fate must have intended and Hollywood would have
scripted, the team that had dedicated its season to its tragically
lost teammate would face none other than the team that
had built its enduring legend in part on dedication to a fallen
teammate – George Gipp's Fighting Irish.

Notre Dame came to Miami ranked No. 4, with 11 wins of
their own but one loss to go with them.

*It seemed like you had forever between the end of the
season and a bowl game. Our last game was November, and
we didn't play until January. We had finals in there, and
then we practiced at CU for a week or so. Then we'd go
down to Miami. That took some adjusting, both about the
move, but also diabetic adjustments.*

*During the regular season, I had a set schedule. I knew
every Monday we would be on the field for two hours and it
would be a light practice. So I knew how to eat and how
much insulin to take. I knew Tuesdays and Wednesdays
would be our hard practices, so I would eat more and take a
little bit less insulin, because I used more energy. Thursday
you tapered down, finalized your game plan. Friday was*

*either a travel day or a really light day.*

*So I had a set schedule of knowing what to eat and how much insulin to take for every day of the week. It took a long time to be comfortable and to have fine-tuned those.*

*I had to have a completely different regimen during finals. As a college student and a diabetic, you don't just stay up all night, cramming for finals. You have to figure out HOW you stay up all night, a lot for the snacking. You're more fatigued because you aren't getting enough sleep, and it affects your metabolism, which affects your blood sugars.*

*So I had one regimen for the season, and another for finals. But we'd never been to the Orange Bowl so I didn't know what the heck to expect when we got down there. And it wasn't as if I could go up to any coach and say, hey coach, are we going to have a really tough practice tomorrow? As much as I had educated them and as much as I was a leader of the team, there were times the coaches didn't even know. Those were some of the more difficult challenges I had.*

*Another factor was the humidity and the heat of Miami. You use a lot more energy in 90 degree weather with 90 percent humidity than you do when it's freezing in Boulder. It's not the fact that you can't handle it as an athlete or your body can't handle it, it just changes how much energy you use, and all of that factors into your blood sugars and how much insulin and how much food. So it was truly a guessing game, minute-to-minute, hour-to-hour adjustments with my diabetes.*

*The other adjustment was the emotional and social.*

*We heard, but we didn't believe it as players, that we were at a disadvantage because it was our first national championship game, whereas Notre Dame had been in these situations before.*

*We didn't believe that. We said, we're a better team. We're going to practice hard. We've got great athletes.*

*But what you forget is we're still kids. We're still really young men who are really, really excited to be here. We were mature enough to say, 'We're really excited to be here, but that's not going to take away from us wanting to win the game.'*

*But there's a big difference between wanting to win the game, and successfully preparing to win the game. And I think that fine line was very tough for us as a team.*

*We had beaten teams that were ranked higher than fourth that year. We looked at them on film, and we weren't awed by them. The part we didn't understand was how to deal with being away from home that long, having the extra pressures of your friends, your girl friends and your family all asking for your tickets and your time.*

*Everyone was excited and wanted to share their excitement with you. We all, as players, were tired after two and half weeks from the pressure on us before the game even started.*

*I make this point whenever I talk to young diabetics, especially ones who want to play athletics: It's important that as a diabetic, when you're tired, you're worn out, and you're blood sugar is coming down, it's not the time to go to your*

*coach and say, 'Hey, Coach, I need to stop. I need a Coke. I*
*need some Gatorade. Can you give me a couple plays?'*

*You need to set the stage and let people know the*
*reasoning behind making those comments. The natural*
*inclination's gonna be, "This guy is trying to get out of this*
*drill." That's where the fine, delicate line comes in, between*
*punishment and pushing someone harder to become*
*stronger and better, and as an athlete, not using your*
*diabetes to get out of hard work.*

*It could happen at any time, not just preparing for a*
*bowl game after the season ends. But the unpredictable part*
*was more likely to happen then, because the coaches were*
*afraid that with finals, with traveling, with extended*
*curfews in Miami – all those things – we better make sure*
*this guy is staying in shape.*

McCARTNEY MOVED his players from their beachside hotel to an
undisclosed location on New Year's Eve.

"I believe a lot can happen in the last 24 hours to help
prepare a guy for the game," he told Denver sports writers. "I
think each guy has to do that within the framework of his
responsibilities. He has to think through different situations he's
going to find himself in, and make the necessary adjustments,
whether he's a coach or a player."

There were no Gipper-like speeches planned or delivered.
In fact, McCartney said, "I've not mentioned Sal's name to our
squad."

But on game night, as Colorado's players arrived in their Orange Bowl locker room, they found Sal Aunese's No. 8 jersey and helmet in a locker reserved for his memory and honor. The message had been sent another way. All that remained was to beat Notre Dame, which was a two-point favorite even though Colorado was ranked No. 1.

One of the key individual match-ups, ballyhooed in the sports pages for days leading up to game day, and highlighted in pre-game network television previews, was the anticipated battle between Notre Dame nose guard Chris Zorich and Colorado's red-shirt sophomore center.

*There was a lot of build-up. One article was basically, the sensitive poet versus the tough street kid from the South Side of Chicago. It was almost comical, especially after I got to know Chris in the years to come.*

*He was billed as this tough kid who didn't know who his dad was, who lived with his mom in an apartment, and was going to Notre Dame – the classic hard-luck kid who had made good despite all kinds of adversity.*

*Talk about a contrast. My mom and dad were still married. Dad was a CEO who went to Stanford. He's highly educated, has a master's degree. Mom's an artist and a teacher. I'm an English major, and "philosophical." The only thing they left out was my diabetes, which was fine with me.*

*I had never met Chris. He was just this guy who was*

*a good player on the other team in a big game. He has huge*
*biceps, and he had this big persona: smashmouth. But his*
*game was just the opposite. His game was all about speed.*

WITH A national championship at stake, Jay thought of little else.
But presented with the opportunity to show Notre Dame what
kind of player it had passed up a few years before, he did not
disappoint himself.

"Buffs interior linemen (center Jay Leeuwenburg and
guards Joe Garten and Darrin Muilenburg) effectively negated
All-American nose tackle Chris Zorich," wrote B.G. Brooks in
the *Rocky Mountain News.* "He had one tackle in the first half."
And one more in the second half.

The game, however, was another story. Colorado domi-
nated the first half but failed to score. Kicker Ken Culbertson was
wide left on a 23-yard field goal attempt. Eric Bienemy fumbled
at Notre Dame's 15 as he attempted to switch the ball from one
arm to the other in the open field. And Jeff Campbell, who held
on placekicks, was stopped short as he dove for the end zone at
the end of a fake field goal after Notre Dame had stuffed three
straight plays in a classic goal line stand at its one-yard line.

McCartney has replayed that night in his mind more than a
thousand times, and holds himself responsible for what followed.

"We completely outplayed them in the first half, and we
didn't score. Then in the second half, they outplayed us. I didn't
give our players what they needed at halftime. They needed real
leadership to put that half in perspective. We were the best

team, and when you have the best team, you have to win the game. I'll always live with that."

Shut out but tied at the half, Notre Dame scored twice in the third period, the backbreaker a 35-yard run by Rocket Ismail, the other with a minute and a half left in the game after driving for almost nine minutes. Colorado's storybook season ended in defeat, 21-6.

"Rocket said there's something mystical about Notre Dame," Irish coach Lou Holtz said after the game. "And I agree with him."

It was the last thing Jay ever wanted to hear.

*At the end of the game, to a man, we felt we had the better team. We felt like we had more talent – that we had outplayed them, but lost on the scoreboard. It was the first time that had ever happened.*

*Truly, it was one of the few times we got out-coached at halftime. They made adjustments, and we said, "You know what: We hold onto the ball and make some kicks, and we're fine." They made some adjustments that we weren't prepared for, and we lost.*

*That was one of the most sickening feelings we, as a group, had ever had. And that night, in the locker room, we said, "We're going to be back here next year, and we're never going to let this happen again."*

*It wasn't like we were going to get up and make promises as a team right then. It was the guys that played, who* had that just sickening feeling in their gut, that said to each other, "We never want to have this feeling again, and we know that the guys that are the core of this team are going to be back." That was the commitment we made that night.

Little did we know it was going to be against Notre Dame again.

# CHAPTER 6

# NATIONAL CHAMPIONS

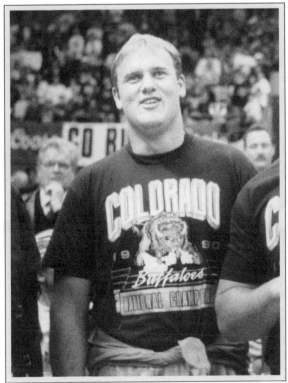

Photo courtesy of Rocky Mountain News

*"After the game there was partying in the hotel,"*
*Jay says of the Orange Bowl victory over Notre Dame.*
*"I remember being just so tired that I didn't*
*participate in the festivities."*

VOWING TO return to the Orange Bowl and play again for a national championship the next year was an understandable, even predictable response from a bunch of macho young men who felt the emptiness of unexpected defeat. That promise to themselves, though, proved easier said than done.

In the season opener, the first-ever Disneyland Pigskin Classic featuring No. 5-ranked Colorado against No. 8 Tennessee, the Buffaloes twice held 14-point leads in the fourth quarter. But when time ran out at the end of a 25-yard pass play that would have moved Tennessee into game-winning field goal range, CU had barely held on for a 31-31 tie.

A disappointing start, but not too disappointing. "You can't say it was almost like a loss," quarterback Darian Hagan rationalized, "because it wasn't a loss."

But after a narrower-than-expected 21-17 win over unranked Stanford in the home opener – ominous in itself for its unexpected closeness – Colorado again blew a two-touchdown lead. This time it was against 20th-ranked Illinois, and this time it resulted in a loss, 22-21.

Three games into their vindication season, Jay and his mates were 1-1-1. National champions? These Buffaloes had barely stayed in the Top 20.

"This takes us out of contention," Bill McCartney lamented to reporters after the Illinois loss. "Last year," mused defensive tackle Gary Howe, "when something unusual happened, it usually went our way. Now it's going the other way, and it's making for a hard season."

The "unusual" pendulum would swing back Colorado's way a few weeks later, but in the gloom of such an uninspired encore, no one could have imagined, or believed, just how.

*We were all looking down the road when the 1990 season started. It was a given that we were going to win. But we had lost some of the focus and some of the attention to detail. We didn't have some of the hunger we had before.*

*We still had that feeling of, "Dammit. We should have been national champion. We did outplay them!"*

*In your mind, as a player, you say subconsciously, 'well, if' and 'well, but.' We looked to blame others instead of ourselves.*

*When we tied Tennessee, we made excuses. It was the weather, and we didn't have this guy and we didn't have that guy. Then we barely beat Stanford. We were rusty, but we won. By then we were struggling.*

*After we lost to Illinois, it was, "OK. There's no chance at a national championship. So we've got to go one game at a time because we'll be damned if we're going to lose the Big Eight championship." Because that was always our first goal.*

*We didn't start getting excited about the potential of being anywhere near the national championship until the last two weeks of the season. There were no guaranteed bowl bids except for conference champions. If you won the Big Eight, you knew you were going to the Orange Bowl. But you had no idea who you'd be playing.*

*Because there were only seven conference games when it was the Big Eight, we played four non-conference games, instead of the three they play now, to start the season. And the Pigskin Classic was considered an extra game. So we still had two games before the Big Eight schedule started.*

MCCARTNEY CREDITS feisty little Eric Bienemy with turning the season around, and doing it without even touching the ball. It was late in the third period of Colorado's fourth game, at unbeaten and then 22nd-ranked Texas. The Longhorns were leading, 19-14, and were driving toward another score.

"I was down around the 20-yard-line, following the play," McCartney recalls. "And all of a sudden I hear this commotion back on our sideline. I had no idea what was going on. I looked over my shoulder, and Bienemy has the whole offensive unit in a huddle around him, and he's grabbing them by their facemasks and yelling at them, and I'm wondering what the heck is going on.

"Then the third period ends, and the teams have to go to the other end of the stadium. The Texas offense runs to the other end of the field, and their fans are standing and screaming. Meanwhile our defense is starting to walk to the other end. They've obviously got us back on our heels. We're about to be toast.

"Next thing I know, our whole offense runs onto the field and stops our defense. And they all get in a huddle, and there's more commotion. I've never seen anything like this in all my years of coaching. I never saw it again. The attitude was, if we have any hope of playing for a national championship again, we have to win this game."

When play resumed, the defense held Texas to a field goal. On the next series, the offense sliced through the Longhorns' defense as it had not done the previous three quarters, and scored quickly. For the first time, Texas went three and out on its next possession, and the Buffs offense scored again. Colorado won, 29-22, the first of ten straight victories.

*Our last non-conference game was at home against Washington. They were ranked 12th –the fourth Top 25 team we had played in five games to start the year. We won 20-14. So we were 3-1-1 going into the big Eight, and you could argue we were only two points away from being 5-0.*

*Our first game in the Big Eight was at Missouri, and one of the things my folks did, being from Missouri, was they chartered a bus for all their family and friends, and they bused to Columbia when we played there.*

*That year they printed up T-shirts that read "Buffalo Breeders" and had one for everybody. So you had 50 people at the game with these T-shirts on, and it was always such a hoot and so good to see everybody after the game.*

*But after that game, nobody from Missouri – my friends – wanted to talk to me. They were just beside themselves over the way the game ended.*

*Missouri had gone ahead 31-27 on a long pass with less than three minutes left in the game. We got the ball on our own 12, and Charles Johnson got us down to their three on a pass to Jon Boman with about 30 seconds left. CJ was playing quarterback because Darian Hagan was hurt.*

*Everybody was scrambling to get in position for the next play, and the clock was running, so CJ spiked the ball. Then we ran Bienemy up the middle, but he didn't get in. So we called our last timeout. It was all pretty frantic, and somehow the down marker didn't get changed. It still had 2nd down.*

*We went over to the sideline, and we're over there talking about what we're going to do. Mac was saying, "We do this on second, this on third and this on fourth down."*

*I know I said, "We can't do that. That will be fifth down."*

*And I remember Mac saying, "I'm the coach. I do the coaching. You're the player; you play. And this is what we're doing." So I was convinced I was wrong.*

*We ran Bienemy, just the way Mac planned it. And*

*when he didn't get in, CJ spiked the ball again, just like Mac told him to.*

*And then on the last play of the game, CJ went right over me. I don't know to this day if he got over the goal line on fifth down. He was right over me. It was really close.*

*They made us come back on the field to kick the extra point, or at least snap it and take a knee. The only people who came back out on the field were the 11 players that were part of the play.*

*They had the six officials run off the field with us because people were hysterical. I truly thought there was going to be a riot. We're running off the field, and not only do we have the officials running with us, we've got police officers, too. So we've got two rings of protection.*

*And then this irate fan from Missouri comes right up to us and throws a beer bottle, and it hits a police officer in the head and knocks him down. I thought the guy was going to die – the guy who threw the bottle, not the policeman.*

*It was insane. Besides the fact that someone would do that to an officer, then to have the officers just brutalize this guy – I thought, "Get me the hell out of here." If they would do this to a cop, what would they do to me?*

*I remember talking to Gerry Dinardo, our offensive coordinator, about the way the game ended on the plane ride home. I remember asking him, "Gerry, did you know?"*

*And he looks at me, and says, 'Jay. It's MY JOB to know what down it is. Do you think I knew?' So he knew. But what could he do?*

THE ROUTE back to the Orange Bowl went through Nebraska in 1990, meaning CU and Nebraska would play in Lincoln, not Boulder. More than two decades had passed since the University of Colorado had won a football game in Lincoln. It was 1967, two years before the oldest players on the 1990 team, including Jay, were born.

McCartney decided the waiting challenge called for an extreme motivational measure.

"Typically we'd finish practice on a Thursday, and we have about a 15-minute team meeting and we'd announce the travel squad. Then the players could do whatever they wanted, work out in the weight room or rest up or whatever. This week, I told the team I wanted to meet for three minutes the next day with each and every player on the team.

"Nebraska has traditionally called its defensive unit the "Black Shirts." But black is our color. So we made up T-shirts that read: "The Real Black Shirts." I told every player to wear their shirt on the plane to Lincoln, because when we land and the TV cameras are there and they get pictures of our players walking off the plane wearing shirts that say "The Real Black Shirts," it'll send a tremor through the whole state. In effect, we were calling them out."

*We go into Lincoln and it's sleeting the whole game, and the temperature's dropping all through the day. It's just miserable. Truly, it was the coldest I've ever been while playing football. You're literally soaked to the bone.*

*Eric fumbled the ball four times in the first three quarters. Two were fumbles at the goal line, going in. And you're going, that's 14 points! We were so mad as an offensive line. We felt like we should be dominating this game.*

*We all knew what a competitor Eric was. Everybody in the huddle knew he was hurting worse than any of us. He came into the huddle and said, 'Give me the ball. I'm going to help you win because I owe it to you.'*

*And then what happened is, we scored four times in the fourth quarter to win. All four scores were Bienemy runs. That's the kind of competitor he was.*

*The thing I'll always remember about winning at Nebraska is going into the stands after the game. We had a great following, probably 3,000 fans. As a team we would always go into the stands and thank our fans for coming to the away games.*

*This one was extra special because we knew we had just pretty much guaranteed we were going back to the Orange Bowl. We still had two games left, but this was the one we had to have. After this, there was no way we were going to lose either of those other games.*

COLORADO'S RETURN to Miami set up the perfect bowl pairing, a rematch of the previous Orange Bowl. The Buffs would come in ranked No. 4 in the nation, and would again play Notre Dame, No. 1 this time, with the national championship at stake.

In a reversal of fortunes that only athletic competition can produce with such sweet irony, it was Notre Dame who this time outplayed Colorado yet lost, by the barest margin of a blocked extra point, 10-9. The Fighting Irish kept themselves from winning with five turnovers and two missed field goals, the final self-inflicted blow a clipping penalty in the last minute that nullified a 91-yard punt return by Rocket Ismail that would have been worth a pivotal six points.

Still able to remember the feeling from the year before, Colorado felt no sympathy and no reason for apology, fifth downs and late flags notwithstanding. If anything, the Buffaloes were a bit ticked when, after the dust from all the bowl games had cleared and they had been voted No. 1 in the national sports writers poll, they were forced to share the national championship throne with Georgia Tech, anointed over them in the vote by major college coaches, at least one or two of whom will forever be suspected of casting spiteful ballots that succeeded in denying Colorado that poll's crown.

Years later, after he had retired from coaching, McCartney was inducted into the Orange Bowl Hall of Fame. Lou Holtz, his adversary on the other sideline during both Orange Bowl classics, attended the induction luncheon. "The scar on the back of my guy's leg is finally going away," McCartney teased, reminding Holtz of the penalty flag. "If you're guy got clipped on that play, he had his helmet on backwards," Holtz retorted with a smile but without even a pause.

No one disputes the flag in Colorado, of course. Rather, the burning question of that Orange Bowl, one that still flickers in the hearts of Colorado's most fervent fans, who remember the game as if it had been played just days rather than years ago, is why McCartney punted to Ismail in the first place.

*We had the ball inside the 50, and our punter, Tom Rouen, punted the ball deep into the end zone. But we got called for holding, so we had to re-kick. They dropped us back ten yards, and Mac never told him to switch his strategy.*

*So Tom tried to kick it through the end zone again. He kicked the same darn kick, but that 10-yard penalty made it to where Rocket could run it back.*

*I snapped for both of those punts. I remember running down the field – I was nowhere near him – and seeing the flags as soon as they were thrown. I said to myself, clip. I honestly never had any doubt. I knew there was no doubt I wasn't going to catch him, but I knew it was coming back.*

*Winning that game was my biggest thrill. DC, my high school coach, was at that game. And so were my parents and my brother. It was THE highlight for me.*

*Truly, the tables were reversed from the year before when we outplayed them and lost. This time, we were outplayed, but won. Almost unanimously, the guys who played in the two games will say the same thing.*

*After the game there was partying in the hotel, and somebody pulled the fire alarm. There was pandemonium. I remember being just so tired that I didn't participate in the festivities. I remember talking to DC, and talking to my parents and my brother, then just going back to my room and drinking some water.*

*Nebraska played Georgia Tech in the Fiesta Bowl, and Tech beat them by a larger margin than we had beaten them. But we had beat the hell out of Nebraska when we played them; literally, like six of their starters were hurt in that game. Our feeling was Georgia Tech didn't play the same Nebraska team. They were missing players, and we felt like we had broken their spirit.*

*We don't talk about that it was a shared national championship, even though it was.*

# CHAPTER 7

# INGHER

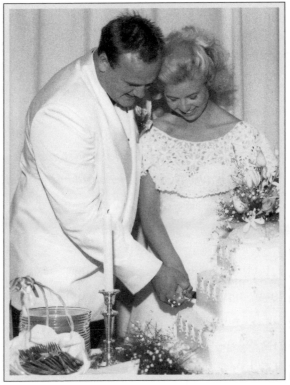

Photo courtesy of Jay and Ingher Leeuwenburg

*"Why do you want to marry my daughter,"*
*asked Fred Bowden.*
*"I cannot imagine my life without her,"*
*Jay answered.*

*"Putting off college for a while? Just graduate
and not ready for what the world has to offer?"*

SO BEGINS the Rail Europe sales pitch, online. "Clearly," it goes
on, "the thing to do is get a rucksack, buy the Eurail Youthpass
and take off for a while.

"If you're under 26 on the first day of travel, you can get a
2nd Class rail pass on the cheap and visit up to 17 European
countries (whether they border each other or not)."

And thus, while the Colorado Buffaloes were winning their
first national championship in school history in the 1991 Orange
Bowl, Ingher Bowden was in London, about to begin the $4-a-
night hostel tour of Europe via her Eurail pass. She was totally
oblivious to CU's success even though she had attended high
school in Loveland, Colorado, a short drive from Boulder.

Ingher was 19 and taking a year off from Rensselaer Polytechnic Institute, where she attended day classes, and nearby Russell Sage College, where she took night courses, a combined load of 24 to 28 credit hours a semester.

"My grandmother was born and raised in New Zealand," she starts the story of her personal odyssey. "She had a brother who lived outside of London and his kids were in London. My mom had been in contact with her cousins.

"I had reached that point in time in college where a lot of kids go abroad to study. I wasn't sure what I wanted to do, but I decided, 'you know what, you're young.' So I took leave from RPI. I just said, 'I'm going to take time off.' I didn't go through their study abroad program or anything like that.

"I said, 'Let's start in London.' My mom's cousin Jennifer is an exceptionally intelligent woman, well-traveled. I decided I'd go spend some time with Jennifer, and see if I liked any of the educational programs there. If I decided that wasn't the thing to do, she was the perfect person to get me going on doing Europe – do the Eurail/hostel kind of thing on my own. Jennifer's a blast – so bright, and she's been all over the world many times over.

"I looked at schools, but I didn't like the programs that would be available to me as an American citizen. So I decided, 'I have X amount of dollars. I'm going to buy a Eurail pass. And I'm going to travel. When the money runs out I'll go home or find a job.' I had sold my car and had tuition money. The deal with my parents was I had to check in once a week by telephone."

The transition from 1990 to 1991 was a historic time for the world. The Berlin Wall had been toppled and the Cold War won

– without thermonuclear obliteration or even superpower combat – just 13 months earlier. Communist rule was ending in Hungary, Poland and Czechoslovakia, and the Soviet Union was beginning to disintegrate. "Operation Desert Storm" became a familiar name overnight as American troops began the liberation of Kuwait from invasion by Saddam Hussein's army.

"My trip started during the first Gulf War," Ingher explains, "so the Eurail pass was limited for me. There were places I could not go as an American citizen.

"It was interesting to be in Europe. I don't speak either language real well, but I read French and German at the third grade newspaper level, enough to get some insights. The European view on the first Gulf War was very different than I had been hearing from home."

Her travels took her to Paris and The Louvre, to see the Mona Lisa; to Rome and The Vatican, where she was hailed from across St. Peter's Square by someone she had met in Helsinki; and, finally, to Athens, where her adventure took an unexpected twist.

"There were no trains to Athens because of the Gulf War," she recalls. "But part of the Eurail pass is some flights. I was leaving Prague, and I called my parents from the airport and told them I really wanted to go to Greece.

"I said, 'I'm almost out of money. I'm leaving on the night flight, so I should arrive in the morning. I'm going to tour around for a couple days, then go back to London. But if I like Athens, I'll find a job and stay for a while.'

"On the flight I met a gentleman who was looking for an

English-speaking nanny for his young son. He wanted his young son to learn English. After a couple days in Athens, I gave him a call. And then I spent time as an English-speaking nanny."

INGHER RETURNED from Greece to a one-semester internship in sports medicine at the University of Colorado that had been arranged through RPI before she left for Europe. She would be a student trainer with the football team, then return to RPI in January 1992 to complete her undergraduate degree – in three years.

She intended to become a doctor, though she had not yet chosen a specialty.

"One thought was orthopedics," she says, "because I loved being in the competitive environment of sports. That's one reason I wanted to do an internship as a trainer. Forensic sciences had always been an interest, too."

As Ingher Bowden pursued her dream on the CU sideline that late summer and autumn of 1991, Jay Leeuwenburg was chasing his across the playing fields of the Big Eight and assorted other universities who were on CU's schedule that year. The coming season, he believed, was his chance to secure his future in the National Football League.

Neither could nor would have guessed that their dreams, as different as doc and jock, would soon intersect. At that point, finding their life partner was the last thing either of them expected, or even wanted.

"You had two very head-strong, ambitious, confident

people," Ingher says. "And young. We were very young. And very ambitious. We had our own ideas individually of where we were going to go. We both had sworn we were never going to get married.

"He's a senior, bigger than life on campus. I know I'm there for six months, there to do an internship. I'd already left home, traveled Europe. I should be responsible and get my degree; finish things up. And he still had a long-term girlfriend who was still semi-in-the-picture."

*I had set the goal for myself going into my senior year that I wanted to be the best center in all of college football. I had made third-team All-American the year before, and all-Big Eight. I told myself there was no reason I shouldn't be the best center in all of college football.*

*She was on the training staff so I'd see her every day. I thought she was attractive. At first I just flirted, kind of joked around with her – nothing extremely serious.*

*I asked her for her phone number, and she wrote it down and gave it to me. I lost it, so I didn't call her.*

*Then I went through the same song and dance again, and she gave me her phone number again. And I lost it again! I truly lost it twice.*

*At this point she is getting a little ticked off. You know, like are you just pulling my chain, or what? I asked her for it again, and she said, 'If you don't call me this weekend, I'm not going to give you another chance. I'm not*

*going to wait around for your sorry butt.'*
*I called her about 9:30 on Friday or Saturday night. I'll*
*never forget her greeting. 'If you're such an athlete,' she said,*
*'then you should understand the rules of baseball. It's three*
*strikes and you're out, and you've already got two strikes.'*
*I've been living with two strikes ever since.*

ASKED WHAT attracted her to the young man she eventually married, Ingher answers with a list of the qualities that quickly includes the traits that enabled Jay to make "Yes I Can!" the words that best sum up his life.

"I tease him all the time that I am a sucker for a great smile," she begins. "He's got that brightness in his eyes every day, that smile that tells you he's got the world by the tail and life is going to be fun. He's also the most uninhibited person I have ever met.

"His strength, and his detriment, are the same thing. He is very confident in who he is. He's not going to be stopped. And that's very threatening to a lot of people, like a lot of the coaches in the NFL.

"Jay's dad and I are very similar, those engineering minds. The numbers will map it out; everything is black and white. Jay is more like his mother, that artist mentality.

"He wants to make the square peg fit in the round hole, or vice versa, and his dad and I are saying, 'The math doesn't work.' And Jay says, 'Bull! I'll make it work.' And you know what? Jay has always made it work.

"Most people like things very concrete: Tuesday follows Monday. But Jay is willing to say, 'That doesn't work for me today. I'm going on to Wednesday.' And it works! You look at him and you want to say, I don't get it; he's driving me nuts.

"Jay lives in the present. There's no past, and he does not plan for the future. That's just not who Jay is. I think a lot of us live with, 'What's going to happen tomorrow? Shouldn't we be planning ahead? Is there a long-term goal here, honey?' But Jay is Jay, every day – strong, secure and confident. He just moves right on."

There is no better example of Jay's stubborn refusal to be stopped than his senior season at CU. He broke his right hand in practice, just three days before the Buffs were to play his dad's alma mater, Stanford, when he caught his ring finger under teammate Joel Steed's face mask.

Everyone assumed he would be unable to play for at least a few weeks. Even Jay thought it was hopeless when he first felt the pain. Team doctors fitted him with a padded cast that exposed three fingers, but he had no control of the ball when he tried to deliver it to the waiting hands of quarterback Darian Hagan.

"The doctors said he's not going to be able to use that hand for some time," Dick Leeuwenburg recalls. "I thought, 'Here we go again. It's the foot thing all over again.' But he just centered with the other hand!"

That might not sound like a big deal to some. But Gary Barnett likens Jay snapping left-handed in a major college football game to "going from being a right-handed pitcher to being a left-handed pitcher in the major leagues."

The ex-lineman in Jay's dad ponders the comparison at first as if it might be an exaggeration, then concedes, "It's a pretty substantial feat Jay pulled off. You take these things you've been doing for years, and all of a sudden it's the mirror image. It's not just the hand. It's the feet. It's everything; everything's coordinated."

Bill McCartney's take on it is unequivocal. "What ultimately happened isn't even possible."

And then McCartney explained what he means. "The center exchange has to be perfect every time. The quarterback can't be worrying about whether or not he'll get the ball, or whether the timing will be right. It would distract his thinking. The center and the quarterback have to be like one. It takes time and a lot of practice to develop that rhythm."

McCartney said he left it up to Hagan whether or not Jay would start at center snapping left-handed.

"It was the quarterback's decision. When he comes to the line of scrimmage, he has a lot of responsibilities. He has to get us in the right play, in the right formation; and he has to read the defense. And he has 25 seconds. He doesn't have time to wonder about getting the ball; it's what he's going to do with it after he gets it.

"Darian said it was no problem. It wasn't that Jay said he wanted to try snapping left-handed. It was that he could do it."

Jay may have surprised his coaches and teammates, but Dick had seen the left-handed side of Jay many times as Jay was growing up.

"What he'd do for fun, the little smart aleck, is we'd be playing Ping-Pong, and he was so much better than I was, all of a sudden you'd notice he's playing with his left hand just so I can score some points! And he's still winning."

*I would always do little things like that, like setting the goal with the pogo stick. We got a Ping-Pong table, and I would beat everybody in the family too easily. So I thought, how can I make this more interesting? So I started teaching myself how to play left-handed. Then I got to the point where I could beat everyone in the family left-handed.*

*I obviously never knew I was going to end up being this football star. Actually, I wanted to be a better basketball player, because that's what I was playing at the time. So I needed to be as good dribbling and shooting with my left hand as with my right. So I would purposely make things more difficult for myself and try to do them left-handed.*

*Now I wasn't such a masochist that I would let it become no fun or painful. If I was playing pickup basketball with my brother in the backyard and I was starting to lose, I would definitely go back to the right hand. Same thing with Ping-Pong. But I would always do things to make it more challenging for me.*

*So when I broke my hand, I was already able to do things left-handed. I just told myself, 'There's no way I'm not going to play.'*

*After that, anything I would have normally done right-handed, I did left-handed. I tried to take notes in class left-handed. I ate left-handed, brushed my teeth left-*

*handed, shaved left-handed.*

*Fortunately, we had a bye week after the Stanford game, so that gave me a few more days to fix it. I followed Darian to every drill those two weeks. Everywhere we went, I practiced snapping with my left hand.*

*I played two games snapping left-handed, and there really wasn't any problem. We didn't have any fumbles or any penalties because we were out of sync. It was really smooth.*

WHEN JAY reported to summer camp that August, the defending national champions were but a memory. Alfred Williams, Kanavis McGhee, Eric Bienemy, George Hemingway and Mike Pritchard had all moved on to the National Football League. Only three starters returned on offense, Jay alone on the offensive line.

He had earned his degree and could have entered the pro football draft, but had another year of eligibility because he red-shirted his freshman season. He chose to play another year, and true to Gary Barnett's prediction when he was selling his top recruit to Bill McCartney years before, Jay was chosen team captain.

A season-opening victory over Wyoming was followed by a 16-14 loss to Baylor that remains to this day Jay's most frustrating example of a young, inexperienced team, as well as a still vivid illustration of the difference between the Buffaloes of the two previous seasons and the team he captained.

A rout of Minnesota that raised hope that maybe the Buffs were going to be formidable after all was followed by the broken hand and a loss to Stanford. So their record stood at 2-2 as they began the conference schedule with a right-handed center snapping with his left hand.

*The only time I seriously thought about saying I was going to forgo my senior season was when I felt like the National Collegiate Athletic Association was penalizing me for actually receiving my degree in four years. The NCAA made it extremely difficult for me because they wouldn't let me have a second undergraduate major. They told me I had to be in a graduate program in order to have eligibility.*

*I was so mad at the NCAA, and it was so tough to get into the Graduate School of Business at CU, that I almost said it's not worth it. Talking to the NCAA was like talking to a brick wall. Their stance with me was, Well, that's the rule, and we're not going to change the rule.*

*The rule has since been changed.*

*The thoughts going through my head were, Would this be a good move for me? Did I have a realistic shot? What would the perception be? There were guys coming out early at that time, but not in the numbers they do today.*

*I think I made the right decision. All the questions about my size and strength, I think, would have been compounded if I had come out early. As a person, I matured a lot more. It helped me a lot being able to go through the struggles of my senior season. Particularly when I got to the NFL, where every week is a struggle, where every week is extremely difficult.*

*My senior season was extremely frustrating, in that we had played for the national championship in back-to-back years, and I didn't know how to lose. Suddenly, going 7-4 was acceptable, and I had a very hard time with that.*

*I had some very young players around me. I couldn't play for them. But I could try to teach them what had made me successful. It was difficult not to be so demanding and so hard on my teammates that it was detrimental.*

*You forget you had to go through those growing pains yourself. But I still was wanting to be at that elite level, and there was just no way, mentally or physically, some of these players could be there. So that was very difficult for me.*

*One of the games I'll always remember is Baylor. I did the snapping for field goals, and with a minute-37 left in the game, we lined up for a field goal that, had we kicked it, would have put us ahead by four.*

*The rookie guard blocked out instead of in, and Santana Dotson blew through and blocked it. The ball went something like 76 yards the other way. Nobody ran it that far, it bounced and rolled that far. I couldn't believe it. We wound up losing, 16-14.*

*Santana wound up playing in the NFL for many years, at Tampa Bay and Green Bay. He always told everyone he beat me on the play, blocked the kick, and won the game for them. When I was with the Bears we always played Tampa Bay twice a year, so I had to hear about it twice a year. And then when I was with Indianapolis, we always played pre-season and regular season games with Green Bay, so I had four more years of hearing his lip.*

*It was things like that that were just so frustrating my last year at CU.*

*Having said all that, we still ended up winning the Big Eight for the third year in a row. We started 2-2, and finished the season 8-2-1. Then we went to the Blockbuster Bowl.*

MANY ARDENT college football fans are thrilled when their team is invited to a bowl game. To them a bid is validation of their season and their program.

Most coaches see it differently. Unless they're playing for the national championship, or maybe a top five ranking in a New Year's Day bowl, the great reward of a bowl bid is 20 or so extra days of practice toward next season, spring football in December without forfeiting spring ball in the spring.

Bill McCartney took that approach to the Blockbuster Bowl. He abandoned the Wishbone offense that had made Colorado such a power, and installed a pro-style passing offense. It paid off in future seasons, but Alabama took advantage of the learning curve to win 30-25.

"We went to the Orange Bowl two years in a row, and on the big stage with a month to prepare, we weren't putting enough points on the board," Coach Mac explains. "We were the best team; we had the most talent; but we weren't putting distance between ourselves and the teams we were playing.

"I decided we needed to change the offense. Alabama was a better defensive team than we had been playing. I felt we had to change things up if we were going to move the ball against them.

"I also wanted to recruit a quarterback who could throw. I wanted to send a message to the kids we were trying to recruit. And we wound up getting Koy Detmer, who became an NFL quarterback, in our next class."

The Blockbuster Bowl wasn't only Jay's last collegiate game. It also was Ingher's last official responsibility as a training staff intern. She figured it would be the last time she saw Jay, too.

"I went to the bowl game then pretty much got back to Colorado on one plane, and left on another for New York," she says. "Jay saw the opportunity to be drafted and play in the NFL. He wanted to go to the NFL Scouting Combine. So in December, we parted ways."

It was only after Jay played in an all-star game in Tokyo that he tracked Ingher down at RPI. This time he had no trouble with lost phone numbers.

*I spent ten days in Japan, and it was just amazing. It was the perfect trip in every way, except Ingher wasn't there with me to share it. It was the only negative thing about the entire trip. So when I came back, I told myself I never want to go on another trip without Ingher. I didn't think it was too late.*

*So, in the totally romantic way I can be, I called her*

on the phone. I was in California with my parents, and she was in New York. Being an old-fashioned guy, I couldn't ask her to marry me over the phone. So I asked her if she wanted to continue our relationship for a significant, long time together.

The conversation went something like this:

'Do you want to be with me for a really, really, long, long, long time?'

'What are you talking about?'

'Well, you know.' And then there was a pause.

'I don't want to say the words over the phone,' I told her, 'because I don't think that's right. As long as I understand that you understand that we want to spend the rest of our lives together, that's what I'm asking you.'

There was no doubt; we knew we were getting married.

I was very excited, and couldn't wait to tell my parents. My mom fixed this big dinner, a welcome home dinner. I sit down, look at them, and say, 'Mom, dad, I've got some very important news to tell you.'

My dad looks at me, then looks at my mom, then looks back at me. 'Who'd you get pregnant?' he asks.

'No, no, no, I didn't get anyone pregnant!' I answered. 'But I am getting married.'

They looked at each other, as if trying to decide who was going to ask. Finally, my dad says, 'To whom?'

'Ingher,' I said.

They looked at each other and both said, 'Oh, thank

God!' It was only then that I found out they were not very big fans of my previous long-time girlfriend.

I got my first dose of reality not too long after that. I went out to breakfast with Ingher's dad, to officially ask if it was okay with him if I married his daughter. They already knew, but I wanted his blessing. That was important to me.

He hit me with a couple of questions that I had never thought of. It's true what Ingher says about me. Long-term planning is not a strength of mine.

We're sitting there, talking about it, and he says, 'Son, how are you going to support my daughter?'

I said, 'What?'

'Well, what are you going to do if you don't make it in the NFL and you have no money, and my daughter wants to go to medical school?'

I had no answer. I kind of went, 'Whoa! I hadn't really thought about that one, Fred.'

His manner was, you better start thinking about it. You need to grow up a little bit and start thinking about somebody besides yourself.

Then he hit me with the clincher. 'Why do you want to marry my daughter?'

I said, 'I cannot imagine my life without her.'

He said, 'That's all I need to know. You have my blessing.'

# CHAPTER 8

# THE 244TH PICK

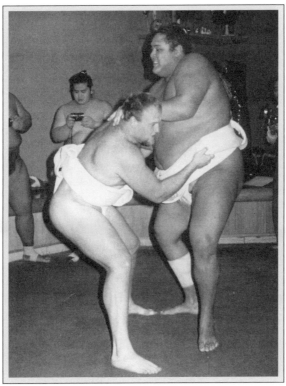

Photo courtesy of University of Colorado

*Jay was invited to every all-star game
after his senior season, but went only
to the Japan Bowl. Sumo wrestling in Tokyo
did nothing to prepare him for the NFL draft.*

AS RUDE awakenings go, the 1992 National Football League draft brought high-flying Jay Leeuwenburg back to earth with the combined force of an illegal chop block and a vicious clip on the same play. What unfolded following the draft blindsided him almost as badly.

Jay had been named a first-team All-American on every post-season team. He had allowed only one quarterback sack, and had been called for only one penalty (on the same play, in a snowstorm in Boulder, he points out) his whole senior season at Colorado.

The year before he had anchored the offensive line of a national champion. In his three years as starting center, Colorado won three straight Big Eight championships; went unbeaten against both Oklahoma and Nebraska; and finished with a record of 30 wins, five losses and a tie.

And he had overcome disabling injury as well as life-threatening illness to demonstrate exceptional durability.

Despite his diabetes and the broken hand, he didn't miss a game, or even a down, because of injury or any diabetes-related complication his entire collegiate career.

Yet when NFL teams began their annual rite of choosing up sides, Bob Whitfield, a 6-foot-7, 300-pound tackle from Stanford was the first lineman chosen. Atlanta took him, with the eighth pick. But at least he was a first-team All-American, too. Then came Ray Roberts, another tackle and a second-team All-American, from Virginia, by Seattle with the tenth pick. Then Leon Searcy of Miami, another second-team All-America tackle, was taken by the Steelers with the eleventh pick.

Eugene Chung, a guard from Virginia Tech, followed at 13th and John Fina, a tackle from Arizona, was next at 27th – neither one even a third-team All-American. And then it was on to the Second Round.

Two more tackles, Greg Skrepenak from Michigan and Troy Auzenne from California, were taken 32nd and 49th. Five more linemen, including the first center of the draft, Washington's Ed Cunningham, taken 61st by Phoenix, were selected in the Third Round.

By the time the unanimous All-American center from Colorado finally was chosen, 36 offensive linemen, including six centers, had been drafted ahead of him.

*I had been invited to every All-Star game there was – East-West Shrine Game, Blue-Gray Game, Japan Bowl, Hula Bowl, Senior Bowl. In my arrogance and cockiness at the time, I didn't think those games were that important. (I now know the Senior Bowl is very important to the NFL, because it's run by NFL coaches.)*

*So I didn't go. I chose to play only in the Japan Bowl, because I wanted to go to Japan. But I didn't play particularly well. I saw the sights and sounds and the different culture. It wasn't about playing football; it was about seeing a different culture, about having a good time. And I missed Ingher. I had fallen head over heels in love with her.*

*After she said she'd marry me, I moved to New York to be with her while she finished at RPI. She helped me pack up all my stuff out of my apartment in Boulder, and I couldn't believe what happened.*

*Under a huge mound of junk in my room, mainly clothes, she found both phone numbers she had given to me. She found both pieces of paper with her phone number on them! She thought I had thrown them away, but I had truly lost them.*

*I didn't have a coach in New York to keep me working and in shape. I thought I had it all figured out. I had been on Bob Hope's Christmas Special, featuring the Associated Press All-America team. I had been in Playboy Magazine's college football All-American spread. So I had obviously already proven myself.*

*I went to the NFL Scouting Combine in Indianapolis, but I didn't do very well. I ran well, but I didn't lift well. I was never a weight room fanatic. The only reason I lifted weights was because I knew I had to in order to play foot-*

*ball. So I wasn't that strong. And even though I weighed 278, as a lineman entering the NFL, 278 pounds is deemed undersized. Most teams wanted guys 290 pounds or more.*

*One of the misconceptions about diabetes is that it's hard to gain weight. It would be too stressful for me to gain weight, or be that big and have diabetes. No one ever asked me about diabetes. So I came out of the Combine with the tag 'undersized and weak.'*

*The other rap on me was the reason I did so well in college was that I was the hardest worker. In the NFL, 'hardest worker' means you don't have that much potential. But even with all of that, I was projected to go somewhere between the 2nd and 4th rounds.*

*The first day of the draft, I gave the NFL the phone number where I would be, in Ingher's dorm room. They went through the first three rounds that first day, and I wasn't drafted. I was really angry. I had to wait another day.*

*Fourth round, fifth, sixth – I still wasn't taken! In my frustration, I wound up ripping the phone out of the wall. Literally. I looked at Ingher, and said, 'Ingher, will you still marry me if I become the manager of a McDonald's instead of playing in the NFL?'*

*She said, 'As long as you can afford to put me through med school.'*

*I was OK with that. I thought, 'I don't mind being poor for a couple of years; I'll be set after that. My wife will be a doctor, and I'll be a stay-at-home dad.' Then we got serious, and she told me that wasn't why she was marrying me. And we started re-prioritizing.*

*I was asking myself what the hell I was going to do with my life. At this point, I still didn't think I had been drafted, because there was no way for teams to get a hold of me. A few hours later, someone told us our phone wasn't working.*

*It was while I was waiting to be drafted that I began to realize how the NFL works. You're like a head of beef when you go in there and do those tests. Every team is asking, 'Who is going to be the safest bet? Who is going to be the best investment for this team?'*

*I'm sure the thinking on me was something like, 'Every lineman gets hurt sooner or later. We're viewing him as a center, and they always get nicked up. He has diabetes, and he won't heal as quickly. Why in the world draft this kid when there are all these questions, real or not, about him?'*

*A few years after the draft, after I had established myself in the league, one of my ex-teammates at CU, who had been drafted the year before me and was doing well, told me he asked his team about me before the 1992 draft. 'What do you think about Leeuwenburg,' he asked. 'I played with him in college. He's a really good player.' He told me later that his team told him I would never play on their team because I was blacklisted because of my diabetes.*

*It was a reminder to me that there was still a ton of ignorance about diabetes, and things don't change very fast. It didn't matter that I had made it, and that I could possibly help the team. It was like, 'We're not going to take that chance.'*

*I was finally taken – in the NINTH ROUND. They
don't even have nine rounds in the draft anymore.*

WHEN THE call finally came, it was the Kansas City Chiefs on the
line. Their first-round pick was Dale Carter, a talented cornerback who would be recognized as one of the NFL's elite defend-
ers until off-the-field problems ultimately made him more
trouble than he was worth.

Before the Chiefs made Jay the 244th player drafted, they
also selected a quarterback and a defensive linemen, both of
whom they traded; a wide receiver; a linebacker and one offensive lineman, who was chosen 31 players ahead of Jay. In the
three rounds that wrapped up the marathon draft that was
shortened to seven rounds the next year, Kansas City picked
another offensive lineman and two more defensive players, an
end and a back.

Despite the assurances of every head coach and general
manager when they assess their haul for reporters and sportscast-
ers after the draft has concluded, no team will know whether a
given year's class is a bonanza or a bust for two or three seasons.
And the final verdict is not returned until careers play out.

It can now be said that the talent scouts and player person-
nel directors and coaches of the NFL obviously underestimated
the diabetic lineman from Colorado. A look at the NFL careers
of the 36 linemen chosen ahead of Jay in the 1992 draft drives
home the point:

- Ten never played a regular-season down in the NFL;
- Half of the first 12 linemen drafted played six or fewer seasons;
- Combined, the 36 averaged half of Jay's total time in the league;
- Only 11 matched or exceeded his longevity as a pro; and
- Of the six centers drafted ahead of Jay, only one played in the league as long as he did. The other five averaged 4.4 years.

Jay bucked the diabetes stereotype and bulked up to 305 pounds; started at all five offensive line positions, something few linemen do; and became a Pro Bowl alternate.

The unanimous All-American who wasn't drafted until the Ninth Round missed only two games (not because of anything related to diabetes, but because of an ankle injury) throughout his entire NFL career, which, as proof of his determination, spanned nine seasons – the exact goal he set immediately following the draft.

Of the ten players Kansas City acquired during the two days of the 1992 draft, seven played in a regular-season NFL game, and only three had long careers. One was Jay. The offensive lineman picked ahead of him was one of those who didn't make the cut.

*I was an angry young man after the draft. I asked myself, 'Is this still something you want to do?' It was. I still* wanted to try it. *It never crossed my mind that I couldn't do this; I had the skills.*

*My goal became to play the number of years in the NFL equal to the round I was drafted in, and prove every team wrong that passed on me.*

*I was determined that I was going to make the team. I knew not everybody who is drafted plays in the NFL, even some guys who are taken pretty high. So when it was time to negotiate my first NFL contract, I wanted a clause that provided that, if I made the team and someone taken above me didn't make it, I got their pay level.*

*I was told to go fly a kite. My signing bonus wound up being $20,000. With that I had to move me out of Colorado and Ingher out of New York. I bought her engagement ring, and after that I was able to buy a gas grill. We had no money.*

*The NFL had a rule that you couldn't go to the city of the team that drafted you until June 1 or after you graduated, which-ever was later. I had already graduated, but the league wouldn't change its rule to allow me to go on to Kansas City. While I waited, Ingher graduated, and we got married.*

IN 1992 THE Kansas City Chiefs were pointing to the Super Bowl as summer training camp began. They had made the playoffs for the second season in a row, but had lost in the second round of the playoffs to one of those Buffalo teams that lost four successive Super Bowls.

These were the Marty Schottenheimer Chiefs, featuring seven players who eventually were named to the Chiefs' "40 Years In Kansas City" 40-man all-time team: placekicker Nick Lowery, cornerbacks Albert Lewis and Kevin Ross, defensive end Neil Smith, linebacker Derrick Thomas and offensive linemen John Alt and Tim Grunhard. But it was another player, tight end Jonathan Hayes, who was of particular interest to Jay.

A second-round draft choice from the University of Iowa in 1985, Hayes had entered the draft with a year of college eligibility remaining, rather than staying the extra year as Jay had done at Colorado. Most significantly, Hayes had succeeded in the NFL with the same disease that Jay had managed so successfully from age 12 to his arrival at his first training camp.

Hayes' diabetes did not develop during childhood. Rather, it waited until spring practice before his final season at Iowa to emerge, and didn't reach crisis proportions until halfway through the schedule that fall. By then the Hawkeyes were contending for the Big Ten Conference championship and the automatic Rose Bowl bid that went with it in the pre-BCS days, and Hayes was the leading candidate for first-team All-America tight end honors.

In his book, *Necessary Toughness*, which was published a year after Jay was drafted by the Chiefs, Hayes tells of hiding his condition from team trainers, doctors and coaches until he was hospitalized that December following the last game of the regular season in Hawaii. He also shares his approach to playing in the pros with diabetes, and some of his experiences with teammates.

"I have always been a person who tries to handle problems

on my own, sometimes more stubbornly than I should," he writes of his efforts to ignore his falling weight and rising blood sugar in his last four college games. "But this was a battle I wasn't going to win alone."

Describing his years with the Chiefs, he writes: "Over the years, most of my teammates have known about my diabetes. I don't broadcast it, but I don't hide it either . . . My greatest fear is that my peers will misunderstand my condition and feel pity for me. I don't want to be treated one bit differently because I have to deal with a serious disease."

*After I thought about it a little, I was glad to have been drafted by the Chiefs. I don't think it was any coincidence that I was drafted by Kansas City. Jonathan Hayes allowed that door to be open to me. To my knowledge then, he was the only diabetic to play in the NFL up to that point.*

*He chose to talk about it later in his career when he wrote his book about it. But I never talked to Jonathan about diabetes. Going to training camp and going through it all, we just didn't have conversations about it. Part of it was that I didn't feel the need. I didn't need to seek him out. I was doing just fine with it at that time. My feeling was, never call negative attention to it.*

*Training camp was tough. If Schottenheimer didn't run the toughest training camp, it was tied for toughest: Lots of two-a-days, lots of contact. There was no free agency at that time, so you played with a lot of veterans. If* you were a young guy, the coach wanted to see how tough you were.

Tim Grunhard was being talked about as an all-pro center. I remember a week into camp telling Ingher that I didn't think he was any better than I was. I told her if they were talking about him along those lines, there was no way I wasn't going to make it in the NFL.

After the second week of camp, Dave Szott broke one of his transverse vertebrae. They moved me to left guard and I started all four preseason games at left guard. I had a lot going for me. I was a backup at guard and center, and I did all the long-snapping.

On the Monday after the last preseason game, we're back at the Chiefs' headquarters in Kansas City. Final cuts were that Wednesday. The offensive line coach, Howard Mudd, calls me into his office, sits me down and we go over training camp. "What did you think? How did it go?" Those kinds of things.

One part of the conversation I remember is Mudd explaining to me that they had 13 linemen in camp, and they only kept eight. Other teams kept nine offensive linemen, but the Chiefs only kept eight. They had some decisions to make, he said, but they rated the linemen on skill and versatility, and he rated me their sixth-best lineman.

So that meant, to me, that I made the team. They keep eight, and I'm sixth: I made the team. I went home and told Ingher, "Let's start looking at houses."

BILL TOBIN carried the ball 75 times, gained 271 yards and scored four touchdowns for the 1963 Houston Oilers. He caught 13 passes that year, too, for 173 yards and another touchdown. Decent enough numbers for a rookie, but it's not because of anything he did as a player that he's almost legendary in pro football.

Rather, it's what other players have done in the NFL – players such as Walter Payton, Dan Hampton and Marshall Faulk, whom he scouted, and either drafted or acquired in other crafty ways. He built the Chicago Bears into the dominant team of the 1980s, then transformed the erstwhile Baltimore Colts from moribund transplant to Super Bowl contender in just five seasons after moving to Indianapolis.

His specialty was finding players. As in, "He's a player." Sometimes it was knowing which college star to choose ahead of others – Faulk, for example, instead of either of two heralded quarterbacks, Tennessee's Heath Shuler and Fresno State's Trent Dilfer, in 1994. Or Payton in 1975 after three other teams passed him up. And sometimes it was plucking someone other teams had underestimated – like Jay Leeuwenburg in 1992.

"I had a reputation for going after character guys," Tobin said years later. "I always had a saying, that when push comes to shove, always go with character. I learned this when I was with Dan Devine in Green Bay. Jim Finks had the same attitude in Chicago.

"I had scouted Jay when he was at Colorado. I had a son who went there at the same time. Jay was what I was looking for. He fit the mold we had developed for character, and he was a tough, aggressive, hard-nosed player.

"During the draft, we had him penciled in as somebody we wanted to take. But when you're drafting, you're drafting for ability, but you're also drafting for need."

The Bears had groomed their next center, Jerry Fontenot, so they waited on Jay while they filled other needs. The Chiefs picked him one round before the Bears would have.

"You don't always get everyone you want," Tobin reminds. "So you keep an eye on them and watch to see if the team that takes them makes a mistake and let's them go. That's how we got Steve McMichael with the Bears; New England let him get away. That's how we got Gary Fencik, too.

"As soon as Kansas City drafted Jay, we moved him to the side and said, when Kansas City makes a mistake on him, we'll get him. We brought him in as soon as they released him. He was always what I thought he was, top-notch character, very unselfish, very committed to doing his job, very committed to winning."

*You'd have to ask Carl Peterson, the Chiefs' general manager, or Howard Mudd – somebody besides me – what their motivation was, but they chose to put me on waivers, the 24-hour waiver wire. Any other team could claim me and assume my contract.*

*The normal day to do this at the end of preseason was Wednesday. Kansas City did it with me at midnight on Monday. According to my agent and Bill Tobin, the GM in Chicago, the Chiefs did this in hopes they'd be able to sneak me through waivers, then put me on their practice squad.*

*They apparently were thinking that if anyone put in a claim after that Wednesday when everyone else was waived, they would say my 24 hours were up. But it didn't work. Chicago claimed me.*

*I practiced Tuesday with the Chiefs – technically after being waived, which is against NFL rules. Then I got a call from my agent, telling me I had been claimed by Chicago. I said, "No, I made the team."*

*Kansas City never said anything. Carl Peterson calls me in, explains the situation, and says, "Here's your plane ticket. You're flying out at 7 tonight, and you're expected to be in Chicago at 8 tomorrow morning."*

*Ingher had been accepted to medical school at the University of Missouri-Kansas City. All of a sudden, she was the one who had to get out of our lease in Kansas City, pack up, and get to Chicago. Meanwhile, I had to find a place to live in Chicago.*

*I had never been to Chicago in my life.*

# CHAPTER 9

# LEGENDS

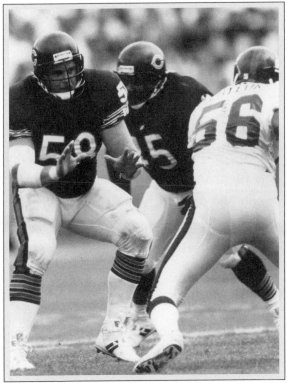

Photo courtesy of Chicago Bears Football Club

*"Here's the bad news," said Bears offensive*
*line coach Tony Wise. "You're not starting*
*at guard. You're starting at left tackle*
*against Lawrence Taylor."*

A GREAT SPORTS town is a special stew: unforgettable athletes, colorful characters and historic figures who are the heart of legend and lore; crazy fans with long memories and vehement differences of opinion, and lots of heartbreaking what-ifs and if-onlys to second-guess; and creaky old bars where the debates live on forever.

Classic ball yards, too, and, of course, championship seasons now and then.

From Papa Bear and Mr. Cub to the Monsters of the Midway and Air Jordan; from the Golden Jet and Harry "Take Me Out To The Ball Game" to Shoeless Joe and the Galloping Ghost; and from Wrigley's ivy-covered outfield walls to the Bleacher Bums beyond them, and Notre Dame, close enough to be claimed as a home team, Chicago has it all.

It is arguably the greatest sports town in America, and everything Jay experienced in four seasons with the Bears only reinforced the notion.

*It was a super town, a fun, fun city to be in. Selfishly, you're treated like a king in that city if you're an athlete. The whole city was just crazy about their sports.*

*My last two years, if it's what I had wanted, I probably would never have had to pay for dinner, wouldn't have had to pay for seeing a movie, or had I gone to a bar, probably wouldn't even have had to pay for a drink.*

*That in itself was unique, but it was never, ever, 'Hey, do something for me.' It was always, 'We love you.' They made you feel like 'It's special that you chose to be here, and as a city we want to embrace you as a city.'*

*I always had the opposite attitude: 'Hey, I'm really excited to play here and thanks for supporting us.' Their whole thing was, 'What are you talking about! It is such a privilege to have you here, and to have you make us feel great as a community to have you around.' There definitely was not that kind of feeling in any other city I played in.*

*You just loved to play in that type of environment. It didn't matter if we stunk or if we were making a playoff run. You always felt like the fans and the community were behind you.*

*I never remember the media ganging up on anybody when things weren't going well. They truly took the game as entertainment. Does that mean they didn't want to win? Absolutely not. But they loved their sports. My recollection is, it was ALL good.*

NOT EVEN the Green Bay Packers, with Curly Lambeau, Vince Lombardi and community ownership, can match the storied history of the football club that plays in the best sports town in America. In the first 84 years of the National Football League and its predecessor, the Bears won more games (646) and more championships (9) than any other franchise.

It all began in Decatur, about 180 miles southwest of Chicago. There in 1920, 25-year-old George Halas who had played the outfield briefly for the 1919 New York Yankees, was hired by the Staley Starch Company to organize a company football team. Halas had played end at the University of Illinois, and on the Great Lakes Naval Training Station team that lost the 1918 Rose Bowl to the Mare Island Marines.

The Staley Starch Company got more than a company team. One year after their formation, the Decatur Staleys, with Halas both coach and player, joined the American Professional Football Association, which, at Halas's suggestion, was renamed the National Football League on June 24, 1922.

A.E. Staley gave the football team to Halas later that year, and paid him $5,000 to keep "Staleys" as the team name for one more season. Halas moved the Staleys to Chicago, won the AFPA championship with a 9-1-1 record, then renamed them the Bears. They quickly became the Monsters of the Midway, nicknamed for the punishing style of play that Halas demanded of all his players.

Chicago's is the winningest franchise in pro football history, and it also has had the most Hall of Fame players. Twenty-six Bears are enshrined in Canton, Ohio, at least one from every decade of the franchise's existence. There's Papa Bear himself and his first superstar, halfback Red Grange, from the '20s; bruising Bronko Nagurski, voted one of the 100 greatest players of all time, and George Musso, the first player to be all-NFL on both offense and defense, among the stars of the '30s; and Sid Luckman, quarterback of four Bears championship teams, heading the best of '40s.

Skip ahead to the '60s, '70s and '80s, and you find Mike Ditka, Dick Butkus, Gale Sayers and Walter Payton.

*The tradition of the Bears is very strong. Part of it is that they keep their great players around the team and involved, even after their careers have ended. Dick Butkus was always out on the field before the game, talking to the guys. Walter Payton was always on the sidelines, like another coach. That was one of the reasons I loved Chicago so much.*

*One of my favorite stories of playing for the Chicago Bears is how I got to know Walter Payton.*

*In college you had, it seemed like, 50 student trainers. So every time you turned around, you had somebody asking you if you needed some water or some Gatorade. Because I was doing the long-snapping on punts, I would be really winded after we'd just had a series of downs and then I snapped on the punt and had to cover the return. I'd get to the sideline and sit down, and in college they knew the routine. They would always come over and give me four or five cups of Gatorade or water.*

*I get to the pros, and that's the last thing I'm thinking of. It may have been the opening game my second year in the league. I was starting and doing all the long snapping on punts, field goals and extra points. It was a hot humid Midwest day at Soldier Field.*

*I come off the field and plop down on the bench, and I'm expecting someone to come over and give me some water or give me some Gatorade. But nothing happens. So I start cussing like a sailor. I start saying, 'Where the h — - is my water?! I need some water! And generally just being a jerk. It's not something I'm real proud of.*

*All of a sudden a hand comes from behind me and gives me a cup of Gatorade. I drink it and I say, 'Give me another one!' I turn around, and it's WALTER PAYTON giving me water and Gatorade. I felt like an ant.*

*As big of a jerk as I was, he would do anything to support you, to help you, to be there on the sidelines. I was so humbled by that experience. In my opinion he was the best football player there ever was.*

*Walter didn't read me the riot act about being a selfish kid. He gave me some water, and let me calm down. Let me feel like the idiot that I was. He didn't say, 'Hey, I'm Walter Payton.' He could tell from the look on my face. It was like, 'Good for you. You were a little jerk, and you should know it.'*

*It came to be that during, every home game, I would have conversations with him on the sidelines during the games. I was able to gain some wisdom and knowledge about football and life. That was a great thrill.*

*It was truly a life lesson. No matter how much you think your stuff doesn't stink, there's always someone out there that you look up to, and when you meet that person, you think, 'I might want to be like him.'*

WHEN JAY reported to the Bears in 1992, the Windy City's sports fans had plenty to cheer, lament, debate and anticipate. The Black Hawks had just lost in the Stanley Cup finals to Pittsburgh. Air Jordan's Bulls were on their way to their second of three straight NBA titles.

Greg Maddux was embarking on a season in which he would win 20 games for the Cubs and win the National League Cy Young Award (even though the Cubs were hopeless, as usual), and the White Sox with "The Big Hurt" were only a season away from winning the American League Central Division.

The Bears under Coach Mike Ditka had won Super Bowl XX in 1986, and the Super Bowl Shuffle (made famous that year by The Fridge, mammoth William Perry) remained popular because the team continued to be a contender through the following six seasons, winning four more division titles. They had been to the playoffs seven times in eight years, including a Wild Card berth in 1991, and had won 90 and lost only 37.

Rich tradition aside, Jay found it unbelievably cool to begin his pro career with the same team for whom his dad had played almost 30 years before. And cooler still that his coach had been one of his dad's teammates, not to mention one of those Chicago legends.

Yes, he was proud and excited. But well short of awestruck.

*I had already played really well against players who were in the league. Chris Zorich was a second-rounder the year before I was drafted, and I felt like I had played pretty well against him for two years in the Orange Bowl. Playing the opponents we played at CU prepared me extremely well.*

*When I was with Kansas City for the pre-season, Tim Grunhard, from Notre Dame, was the starting center. And the Chiefs were saying he was going to be a future Pro Bowler. He was young, probably third or fourth year, and he was a guy they were looking for to be a leader, an up-and-comer, one of the best in the league.*

*I had gotten to a place where I truly felt I was very good at analyzing film and looking not only at my play but at the play of others. And I felt I was as good as Tim Grunhard. There will be lots of people who will say that's a bunch of baloney, that there's no way. But I felt I could do the things he was doing as well as he was doing them, and some things better.*

*That gave me a ton of confidence as I moved to the Bears. I felt that if this is a guy who is supposed to be the best of the best in the National Football League, then this is definitely where I belonged. I felt I should definitely have a spot in the NFL.*

*That probably sounds arrogant. In my mind, there's a difference between being arrogant and being cocky. Arrogant is when you can't back it up. You're cocky if you're really confident and not afraid to say so.*

*When I got to Chicago, there were 25 players still on the team from the Super Bowl champions. Mike Singletary was still there, and The Fridge and Richard Dent, Mark Carrier and Steve McMichael on defense. The offensive linemen were Keith Van Horne, Mark Bortz and Tom Thayer, and the center at the time was Jerry Fontenot.*

*The big news was they had just gotten rid of Jay Hilgenberg, their seven-time Pro Bowl center, because he wanted a million dollars and they wouldn't pay him more than $950,000. The quarterback was Jim Harbaugh; the running backs were Neil Anderson and Brad Muster.*

*I didn't actually start until my second year. But I was in on kickoff returns, and did some punt snaps and some field goal-extra point snaps. After the eighth game, it looked like we weren't going to have a winning season, so I started playing every other series.*

*I would go in for one series for Mark Bortz and one for Tom Thayer, both at guard. They had both been in the league over ten years, all for the Bears because there was no such thing as free agency then. So out of respect, they always had them start. But I got some invaluable experience.*

*I loved playing for Ditka. He wanted tough, hard-nosed guys who didn't bitch or complain, and would go out there and hit you in the mouth. Literally, the more fights you got into, the harder you were trying and the more he liked you.*

*Ditka's whole motto was: "I don't care how you get it done, but get it done. I don't care if you stand on your head, as long as you get the guy blocked." And he meant it.*


DESPITE THEIR playoff appearance 18 months earlier, the Bears of 1992 were a team in decline. Singletary, wrapping up a Hall of Fame career, played his final game in Soldier Field on December 13 that year. His last hurrah was one last taste of the good old days, a 30-6 upset of the Pittsburgh Steelers, who were headed to the playoffs as American Conference Central Division champions.

But not even that was enough to save the head coach's job. Jay's rookie season started 4-3 but ended 5-11 as the Bears beat only the Steelers in their last nine games. On that note the Mike Ditka Era officially ended, with 113 victories and 67 defeats, including six of each in post-season.

Chris Leeuwenburg remembers Ditka's last game as head coach, though not because it was Ditka's last game. It was the first time Chris got to see his brother play in the NFL, and a big moment in Chris's life, personally, too.

"I saw Jay play at least one game in the NFL every year," he says with pride. "His rookie year, I saw the last game of the season in Dallas. I was living in California then, and my work schedule allowed me to get away for a couple days.

"I met my girl friend, who is now my wife – Her name is Anne-Marie, but I call her Anna – and got to see Jay for dinner. He got my room for me in the same hotel the team was staying in.

"The next day I proposed to Anna, and then we went to the game. Jay played the whole second half. Anna and I both had to leave with about three minutes left in the game, to catch separate flights. It was hard to leave. Jay was playing pretty well."

In January 1993 Dave Wannstedt became the eleventh head coach in Bears history. With him came an entirely new coaching staff, and an opportunity for Jay to become a regular in the NFL. In his first start, he got to know perhaps the greatest linebacker in the history of pro football.

LAWRENCE TAYLOR'S story has been told more than a thousand times. Lightly recruited because he didn't start playing football until he was a junior in high school, he went to North Carolina and became an All-American. The second player chosen in the 1981 National Football League draft, he made the Pro Bowl ten straight years beginning in his rookie season.

He became L.T. – the only defensive player in the history of the NFL to be consensus player of the year. He led the New York Giants to two Super Bowl championships, in 1986 and 1990, and was inducted into the Pro Football Hall of Fame in 1999.

L.T. played outside linebacker, and ate left tackles for the appetizer before feasting on a main course of blind-sided quarterbacks. The previously unheard-of combination of a man 6 feet 4 and 240 pounds with the lightning quickness of a blitzing cornerback produced 142 quarterback sacks in 12 seasons.

It turned out, though, that he was human after all. At least twice during his playing days his dependency on cocaine became public, and in 1992 he ruptured an Achilles tendon. He returned for one more season in 1993 before retiring at the age of 34.

*When I went to training camp during Wannstedt's first year as head coach, they told me I wasn't going to be their center because Jerry Fontenot had paid his dues and he was going to be the center. So I had to battle it out for guard. They had drafted a kid out of Kentucky named Todd Perry in the third round.*

*We battled all through training camp. I didn't know if I had won the battle or not, because you learn pretty quickly that it doesn't matter what you think. It's what the coaches think.*

*A coach that I very much enjoyed and loved playing for was Tony Wise. He was line coach for the Bears under Dave Wannstedt. Tony called me up to his office and said, "Jay, I have some good news and some bad news."*

*He didn't give me a choice. He said, "This is the good news. The good news is you're going to start against the New York Giants on opening day for the Chicago Bears. Congratulations!"*

*So I was fired up. I thought, 'Yes! All right! All my hard work had paid off. They saw that I was talented, that I was the player I thought I was.' Everything was the way it should be.*

*Then Tony said, "Here's the bad news: You're not*

starting at guard; you're starting at left tackle against Lawrence Taylor." So my first start in the NFL was at left tackle against L.T.

Tony tried his best to help me get ready to start at left tackle. "I want you to do everything left-handed," he said. "I even want you to wipe your butt with your left hand." I'm remembering my broken hand in college and thinking, 'I've already done this.' But I said, 'That's a great idea, coach.'

It was L.T.'s first game back after his Achilles injury, and I had a great three and five-eighths quarters. L.T. had one assisted tackle.

We were down 10-7 with just under two minutes left. We got the ball on our 20 and were driving down in the two-minute drill to go for the win.

L.T. got me on an outside move. Right or wrong, I think he might have had a little help from some substances on the sideline. He had a different gear that I had not seen the entire game. He went by me, sacked Jim Harbaugh, caused a fumble, recovered it, got player of the game, and they won, 10-7.

One play, and certain members of the community and the media were asking why I was even in the game. That was a true wakeup call to the NFL.

IF ANY defensive player in the NFL rivaled L.T. in his prime, it was the late Reggie White, who retired as the NFL's all-time sack leader with 198.

White's statistical biography points out that he recorded his 100th quarterback sack in his 93rd game – 21 games faster than L.T. – and that in eight years with the Philadelphia Eagles he finished with more sacks (124) than games played (121), the only player to accomplish that feat. It also notes that he was selected to play in 14 straight Pro Bowls (compared to L.T.'s 10); and, most impressively, that 73 different quarterbacks collapsed under the weight of his 300-pound rush.

When told that White had died unexpectedly in January 2005 at the age of 43, Green Bay quarterback Brett Favre said, "He may have been the best player I've ever seen, and certainly was the best I've ever played with or against."

Jay would agree, based on the first taste he got of Reggie White.

*I had to play left tackle for at least four weeks. Troy Auzenne was supposed to be the starting left tackle, but he had torn a ligament in his knee. So I ended up starting the first six games at left tackle. I thought I got better each week. I was feeling pretty comfortable, doing pretty well.*

*Maybe because I was still that confident, cocksure kid, I thought I had a realistic shot of staying at left tackle after Troy got better. But when he came back after the sixth week, I got another call up to Tony Wise's office.*

*"We think you're doing a heck of a job at left tackle," Tony began, "but we don't feel like it's fair to Troy that he's not our starter at left tackle because of injury. So you're not*

*going to be our starter at left tackle. But we don't feel right*
*tackle is doing as well as it should be."*

*So they moved me over to right tackle. I started my*
*seventh game at right tackle. We just happened to be playing*
*the Green Bay Packers. So I got to go up against Reggie*
*White. It's a huge deal starting, and it's a huge deal going*
*against Reggie White.*

*It was similar to starting against L.T., except this one*
*wasn't on the last play of the game, and it wasn't the play*
*that broke the camel's back or anything like that. But there*
*are certain plays that you just remember.*

MOST FOOTBALL fans have the same problem, whether they realize it or not. They don't really understand what they're seeing.

They know the quarterback connected with the wide
receiver for 40 yards, or the running back broke loose for 25, or
that big defensive tackle stuffed the play in the middle or the
quarterback had no chance on that safety blitz. And they
wonder why the offensive coordinator doesn't call that pass play
again, or why they ran up the middle or why they didn't see that
blitz coming.

Too often, the average fan doesn't realize that the running
play that was stuffed at the line is the same one that went for a
big gain the time before, or that the pass that went for 40 last
time was intercepted this time. Most importantly, they have
little or no idea why something worked once but failed the other
times it was called.

Football is so complex, the variables on each play so many, and the players involved so numerous, that it takes a coach or a player, or a former coach or former player, to recognize the subtle differences that decide the success or failure of most plays.

Jay's first encounter with Reggie White is a perfect illustration.

*One of the things that helped me out tremendously is that my intelligence allowed me to anticipate what was going to happen before it happened. I would study defenses and tendencies and specific players, and I really felt like I could anticipate where they were going to go and what they were going to try to do, and that helped slow the game down for me.*

*One of my coaches always said that the key to being a good lineman was to be able to do exactly that, to make it seem like it was almost in slow motion. Once you got into one of those situations where you were reacting and feeling like there was a ton of stuff going on around you, it made it much more difficult. In order to recognize quickly there was a 'game' – that this isn't just a guy rushing upfield – the quicker you can recognize that and pass that off to your tackle or the guy next to you, the better you're going to be.*

*If you get hit by a blitz you didn't see coming, you think, 'Whoa!' and there are guys flying by you. But if I already knew the safety was dropping down and the corner was rolling, that it was coming, then I'm sitting there licking my chops saying I can just pepper this smaller guy.*

*And I think that's what made me more successful than a lot of other people.*

*Against Reggie, I distinctly remember we were around their 20-yard line, going in for a score.*

*On this play the linebacker came up and tapped Reggie on the butt, which meant he was supposed to kick down over the guard and rush over the guard. Of all things, it's called shifting to the Bear defense. They put the defensive end on the guard, so they cover up all three of the interior linemen, and then the tackle goes out and blocks the rushing outside linebacker.*

*Coverages are changing. I've got the linebackers where they're supposed to be. So I call to my guard, and I say, essentially, you've got him. He's moving; you've got him.*

*It was a quick count so they snapped the ball, and I went out and blocked the outside linebacker. The only problem is, the guard doesn't have the end until he physically moves over him. Reggie ended up slanting right into the guard, going off the guard's butt. He went unblocked.*

*It was technically my fault. I knew he was supposed to go right into the guard, but since he didn't actually move, he was technically still mine. So I was credited with giving up one of Reggie's 198 career sacks.*

*It was what I would consider a rookie-type mistake. Even if you know where they're supposed to go, you've still gotta block them where they are. It was my mistake, because I had not played enough football.*

*They were baiting me, and Reggie was a really smart*

*player. He knew I was a young kid, getting my first start at right tackle. So even though he was supposed to move over the guard, he just waited and let me react before it actually happened.*

*I think Reggie was the best player I ever played against. I remember one time we had a third-and-one, where all I had to do was the back-side cutoff. I thought I had perfect position, perfect pad level, perfect everything. It was like hitting a brick wall.*

*He was the strongest man I've ever gone against. He played with such terrific leverage and technique. It wasn't just against the pass; it was against the run and the pass. He was a great player.*

JAY PLAYED the last ten games of the 1993 season at right tackle, then started at his third position in two years, right guard, in 1994. Coming off a 7-9 season, the Bears were not expected to contend in their division. But an unbeaten November left them 8-4 with four games to play.

Every player in the NFL dreams of making the playoffs and winning the Super Bowl. Suddenly, the first of those dreams was within reach for Jay in just his third season.

Trips to Minnesota and Green Bay, both also still dreaming of the playoffs, awaited back-to-back. Making the playoffs would likely come down to winning at Soldier Field against the Rams, who were indifferently playing out their last season in Los Angeles, and the Patriots, who were battling Miami for first place in their division.

The Vikings won in overtime, then the Packers steamrolled, 40-3. In the last game of the season, on Christmas Eve, the offense again produced only three points as New England won despite scoring only 13.

With a lone December victory the week before against the Rams, though, the Bears ended their schedule with a 9-7 record. That tied them with the New York Giants for the last Wild Card berth, and a better record against common opponents gave them the tiebreaker.

Jay's Christmas present was a return trip to Minneapolis for his first taste of post-season intensity.

*When you rank the stress level and intensity of games, opening day is pretty intense. It's your first real game after the pre-season. The intensity and the speed definitely go up.*

*Then the next level comes when you say, 'Okay, we have to win down the stretch to get in.' The last few weeks of a season you have a pretty darn good idea what you need to do. You go through all the scenarios of who you're playing and who they're playing, and what you have to do to get in.*

*You think at the time that it's playoff mentality, but you don't really understand what playoff mentality is until you're in the playoffs. Then it gets kicked up another degree. It's a combination of the teams you're playing are better; the media attention is greater; and the attention to detail, the intensity from the coaches and from the players –*

*the seriousness – it all goes up.*

*We felt very good about going to Minnesota, even though we had lost to them twice. Statistically speaking, we had all these little things going for us.*

*First, it's very rare that a team that is swept in the regular season loses to the same team a third time. Second, the team that got skunked in the regular season historically comes back and wins in the playoff. And third, at least one visiting team always wins in the first round of the playoffs. A visiting team had not won, and we were the last of the four being played.*

NO TEAM was willing to use even its last draft choice on John Randle when he came out of Kingsville's version of Texas A&M. Hoping for a chance to show what he could do, he signed with the Vikings as a free agent before training camp in 1990.

There was no obvious reason to believe he would make the team, and even less cause to think he could become a superstar. Yet he did both, lasting 14 seasons; going to seven Pro Bowls, six of them in a row between 1993 and 1998; and retiring in fifth place on the all-time quarterback sacks list.

Oddsmakers made the Vikings a touchdown favorite going into their third meeting of the season with the Bears. And why not? They had Randle and his career-high 13.5 sacks that season to lead the defense, and prolific Warren Moon running the offense.

Meanwhile, the Bears hadn't beaten Minnesota in three years, losing six straight; hadn't been to the playoffs in three years; and had the lowest-scoring offense of all 12 teams to make the post-season – the only one to finish with fewer than 300 points in 16 games.

Jay's probability omens, however, were right on the money. The Bears offense erupted for 35 points – eight more than its best output of the regular season, and stunned the Vikings, 35-18. Randle finished with a single tackle.

*I was playing right guard and the key matchup for our offense was me against John Randle. He wasn't playing tackle; he was playing what we call a three technique, which meant he was always lined up over the guard. We knew that if we set the formation with the tight end on the right side, that 90% of the time John Randle would be over me.*

*The coaching staff went in saying this is our matchup, and a large portion of our game plan depends on how you do against him. I played very, very well. Part of it was scheme; part of it was that we were able to run the ball. But I also had one of my best games.*

*I did not give up any sacks, any pressures, and I was going up against an all-pro, one of the best in the business at the time. So I felt really, really proud of the way I played. I felt like I was a major factor in our win.*

*Winning a playoff game was the highlight of my pro career. I don't know if I can imagine what it would be like to win a Super Bowl because the feeling you had after being on the road and beating a team, and knowing you played well – I don't know if there's a sweeter feeling in football.*

*It was extra neat because Ingher was able to travel and go to that game. I saw her during the pre-game warm-ups, and was able to go over to the stands and give her a kiss before the game. It was special that she was there.*

ASK INGHER Leeuwenburg what it was like to be an NFL wife, or how she liked being an NFL wife, and her answer will begin with a clarification.

"I always viewed myself as an NFL fan, a fan of Jay's," she declares, "never an NFL wife. I went to football games because I enjoyed watching my husband play football. I didn't go to football games to be seen."

Soldier Field in the early '90s was too antiquated to have a dedicated section for the families of team members, so players' wives were given tickets for seats throughout the stadium. "I loved it," Ingher says, establishing one of many differences between her and any woman whose status as an "NFL wife" helped define her identity. "You were with season ticket holders who had passed them down year after year for generations."

The first game Ingher attended as the wife of a Chicago Bears player will live forever in her memory, though not because of anything Jay did that night.

"Jay had made arrangements for me to go with the wife of another player who was new," she begins. "This was big league. Even though it had been several years since they had won the Super Bowl, this was still the "it" crowd of the NFL. You still had 22 starters from that Super Bowl team. You still had all the money, all the talk, all the walk. And it was Chicago, so we're talking BIG-LEAGUE sports town.

"We showed up to the football game dressed for football – T-shirts, jeans and cowboy boots – and we were ready to order a beer. We had our Wives Passes, to go to the Wives Room. So at halftime we said, 'Okay, let's go check it out.'

"It was August, but there were ceiling to floor minks, and chenille like you could not imagine. Not one person in that room, in our estimation, was dressed for a football game.

"Right there, that set the tone for me. I was thinking, 'I don't fit in. I'm here to watch a football game.'

I wore jeans to every football game after that. In fact, I have a pair of cowboy boots in every color of every team Jay ever played for. So, I guess you can't take the Colorado out of the girl."

Ingher quickly understood the turn her life rather unexpectedly and quite suddenly had taken, and had surprisingly little difficulty making the transition from aspiring medical student to supportive spouse and champion of the unique pro football player who had become her husband.

"Even being married was never a vision I had," she explains, "so all of this was very different. It was never that Jay's career was more important. It was just, 'This is now.'

"It truly is, 'You get one shot.' The opportunities the NFL was going to afford us were only going to happen once. The NFL, like any other part of the entertainment business, is all in the moment. That's one thing we realized as soon as Jay became a starter.

"Sports are different from Hollywood, for example, in terms of entertainment, in that you're never going to have a couple pursuing the same career. So you don't ever have that competition in a relationship."

"Soccer mom" doesn't fit Ingher much better than "NFL wife," but she does have two daughters, Cora and Kate, who keep her on the run with school activities and a variety of lessons that include ballet, horseback riding and swimming.

"We were married five years before we had Cora. We had gotten pretty comfortable with the lifestyle without kids, at a very young age. We had reached the point that if we were going to take that step, as part of married life, we knew we would want to do that while we were young.

"Being the type of people Jay and I are, and the type of parents we wanted to be, or wanted to commit to being, that meant always having a parent at home. Whether that fell to me while he was playing, or whether after football he chose a career that enabled him to be more involved with our children's lives, the NFL provided opportunities and financial security most young couples don't get."

# CHAPTER 10

# CRITICAL IGNORANCE

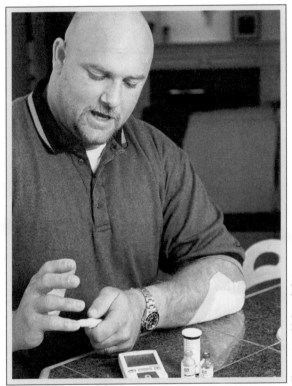

Photo courtesy of Indianapolis Star

*From prescribed medicine to IVs, Jay encountered*
*potentially life-threatening mistakes in the NFL.*
*"We never had a diabetic before,"*
*team doctors and trainers told him.*

ONE FACTOR, more than any other, influences the careers of most NFL players.

It is not natural talent or acquired skill, because only the exceptional make it that far to begin with. It is not desire, though wanting it more than the other guy and refusing to be denied ultimately separates the similarly gifted. Nor is it character, even if it is true that, as coaches are always saying, when the going gets tough, the tough get going.

That factor is injury. For, with the size, strength and speed of the men who play such a violent game, it is not so much a question of IF a player will get hurt, as much as WHEN. And WHAT, too. Ankle? Knee? Shoulder? Back? Head?

This is why Dick Leeuwenburg, when reflecting on Jay's outstanding career, says he was always more concerned with his son as a successful person. "I never got that worked up about this whole football thing," he says. "I never allowed that to be the primary thing in my mind as I thought about my son.

Having played, I knew the next hit could end your career."

Fortunately, Jay avoided that catastrophic collision throughout his nine seasons of pro ball. But that doesn't mean he didn't have to deal with injury, other physical difficulties and the added complication of diabetes.

His first episode began with a back injury. It occurred during an off-season mini-camp between his first and second seasons, soon after Dave Wannstedt took over as coach of the Bears.

*The old training facility the Bears had before they built a new $20 million complex in the late '90s was an old bubble. It was inflated – nothing fancy – and cold. Our weight room was in the middle of this cold facility.*

*I always liked to work out in the morning, and one of the first lifts you have to do are called power cleans. You lift and jerk it up in one motion to your chest. Being in the bubble that had no heat, I hadn't warmed up properly. I tried to do too much weight too soon, and I instantly felt a pop in my back. I just fell to the ground.*

*I iced it, and worked around a little bit, and it didn't feel like it was that big a deal. That was in the morning. Then we had meetings, where I sat for a couple of hours. Then we had two to three hours of field work, where you're out there practicing. You go through all the drills.*

*During the pass protection drill, you're supposed to punch with your hands against another offensive lineman who is supposed to give you pretty good resistance. When*

*I did that, it was like somebody shot me in the back. I fell over and I couldn't walk, but not because I had lost feeling. Something had happened; I just didn't know what.*

*I went in and took a shower, got some treatment on my back, and was told to go home. That was when I realized I couldn't even get dressed. I had managed to get my underwear on, but I couldn't bend down to put my socks on my feet. I was sitting there and couldn't get my flippin' pants on.*

*It was a mini-camp, so we probably had 70 guys there that day. And everyone was making their way out of the locker room because they wanted to get home. It was the off-season. Everybody was in a hurry to get out of there.*

*After seeing 35 or 40 guys walk by and ignore what I thought was obviously a guy struggling, I was starting to get really ticked off. I remember leaning over and thinking, 'OK, I've got to do this. It's going to hurt like hell, but I don't have any choice.' I was almost in tears because it hurt so much.*

*Then this guy stops and says, "You okay? You need some help?'*

*I said, 'Yes. Please. Will you please help me get my pants on?'*

CHRIS ZORICH finished his college career a year before Jay, and was drafted in the second round by the Chicago Bears in the spring of 1991. His last collegiate game was the Orange Bowl rematch of Colorado and Notre Dame, which also was Round Two of Jay Leeuwenburg, All-America center, versus Chris Zorich, All-America nose tackle.

The head-to-head replay, however, never materialized. After seeing Jay neutralize their star player in the first meeting, Notre Dame's coaches positioned Zorich so that he would avoid head-to-head blocking by Jay the second time around.

The strategy freed Zorich to be named the most valuable player despite Colorado's narrow victory. But it didn't prevent the two from tussling on occasion during the game.

What happens at the bottom of a pile is often alley fighting to the power of ten. The grabbing and clutching can get pretty personal, and has the potential to change a young man's voice by several octaves at the high end of the scale.

Such was the case, Jay recalls, on successive plays early in the second Orange Bowl game, as first Zorich then Jay groped and squeezed. Having reached an understanding about such things, they concentrated on football thereafter.

Neither could have imagined that night that they would become NFL teammates within a couple of years, much less how their personal relationship would develop. Intense rivals became improbable friends when the Bears claimed Jay from Kansas City the year after making Zorich their first-round choice in the 1991 draft.

*It was sort of an unwritten rule that, once you reach*
*a certain level in the NFL, you can't maintain game tempo*

*in practice or you'll just burn out. Chris and I took a little longer for that to set in. We were young enough in our careers, and it was our personalities, that we still thought you played the way you practiced. So we were going to practice full speed.*

*It was his job to beat the hell out of me in practice, and my job to do that for him. I knew if I didn't give a hundred percent in practice, he'd be offended. And he knew if he didn't give a hundred percent in practice, I'd be mad. I'd be saying, 'What's wrong with you? I'm supposed to get better."*

*We'd just pummel each other in practice, and we loved each other for it. We would literally get in fights three or four times every practice. These were not kind-hearted, pat each other on the butt, 'good job' fights. We were trying to rip each other's helmets off, and see who was the bigger man.*

*Having said that, Chris became one of my closest teammates. One of the things I most respected about him was that, just as I think I was, he was such a jerk and so competitive, and just so nasty, on the field, but he was one of the nicest guys I ever met, and just a gentleman, off the field.*

*He was the only guy who stopped to help me that day I hurt my back. He knelt down and helped me get my pants on over my feet so I could pull them up. When I was finally dressed, he walked me to my car.*

*Knowing what a humbling position he put himself in, I was so grateful. It was one of those life moments when I wondered if I would have been as gracious in the same situation.*

*That's when I knew what a class guy he was. Not that*
*he was just being nice and it was superficial. He meant it.*
*He was a genuinely caring individual. I will always*
*remember his act of kindness. I get emotional thinking*
*about it even now, years later.*

THE INJURY that left Jay temporarily crippled was diagnosed as a compressed spinal disk. As he explains it, there are disks between all of the vertebrae in the spine. When a disk is compressed, it bulges out. And when it does that, it can press against the nerve that sends impulses to the legs to make them function.

Within days, Jay was participating in a regimen of exercises and physical therapy designed to relieve the pressure and return his spine and back to normal. With that treatment, doctors prescribed medication called a Medrol Dose Pack to reduce the inflammation around the nerve root.

Spine-health.com, an Internet site devoted to providing reliable medical information about a wide range of subjects related to back and neck pain and related conditions, offered an easy-to-understand explanation of the Medrol Dose Pack:

"Oral Steroids, a non-narcotic type of prescription medication, are very powerful anti-inflammatory medications that are sometimes an effective treatment for low back pain. Like narcotics agents, oral steroids are intended for use for short periods of time (one to two weeks).

"Oral steroids come in many forms, but are usually ordered as a Medrol Dose Pack in which patients start with a high dose for initial low back pain relief and then taper down to a lower does over five or six days.

"When used on a short-term basis, there are generally few complications associated with oral steroids. There are, however, a number of potential complications associated with long-term usage of oral steroids. Adverse side effects can include weight gain, stomach ulcers, osteoporosis, collapse of the hip joint, as well as other complications.

"It is important to note that diabetics should not use oral steroids since the medication increases blood sugar . . ."

*I started taking the Medrol Dose Pack, and all of a sudden, my sugars are 500, but I don't know why. I'm slowly increasing my insulin, but I'm saying, 'There's no way I should need this much insulin. What the heck is going on?'*

*If your blood sugar is consistently 500, you're probably headed for the hospital, diabetes-wise. That's dangerously high. I'm not talking occasionally. I was there for a long time, meaning hours.*

*Say I would take a normal insulin dose of 12 units. I would have to triple my insulin level in order not to have a high blood sugar. Whenever you have to do that, you're just scared. You're going, 'This is not normal.'*

*I was conditioned that if I took insulin in that quantity, that would normally kill me. Because if you're going to triple your dose, you're supposed to be having insulin reactions in the worst scenario.*

*After two days of me telling the doctors about this, they say, 'Oh, yeah. One of the side effects is you might have elevated blood sugars.'*

*I'm thinking, 'Really!! You think so?'*

*I'm doing this so my back gets better, because I want to play football. But at the same time, I don't want to have my sugars elevated to a point that's life-threatening.*

SIDE EFFECTS. Before something as routine as an eye examination at the neighborhood Eyeglasses-R-Us shop, patients are routinely asked to fill out a medical information form. Included are the questions, "Are you allergic to any of the following medications?" and "Do you have any of the following?" – with diabetes included in the list that follows.

Such attention to detail, however, breaks down on the sidelines and in the training rooms of the NFL.

The reality of Jay's professional career was that any mistake by team doctors or trainers in treating even relatively minor physical problems had serious consequences. It was up to him to try to prevent these occurrences.

*I naively thought the doctors and the training staff in the NFL would be leaps and bounds better than those I had in college. Meaning, you hear how quickly guys come back from injury, how the perception is there's this cutting-edge technology for these elite athletes.*

*They didn't know anything about diabetes – none of them. I had to do it all over again from scratch. I had to educate every training staff and all the doctors that were the team doctors for all of these football teams.*

*They were asking me, basically, 'How do you do it?' Rather than giving me advice on how to be more successful, I really got the distinct impression that it was,'"So, Jay, how's it going? Tell us about this.' That was a huge eye-opener.*

*I thought I was going to get this reprieve: 'Oh good, I don't have to go back and educate everybody again.' But they were as naïve as everyone else I had dealt with. It makes sense, because there were almost no other diabetic football players. But I would have thought they would have been a little better prepared.*

*One situation happened to me two or three times, so pick a team. One of the problems I started having was I became susceptible to muscle cramps. Pretty severely, to the point that I needed IVs.*

*I was cramping because we were in two-a-days during training camp; I was with the Bears at the time. It was hot as hell, and I lost something like 14 pounds in one practice. I started getting muscle cramps because I was so dehydrated.*

*They put me on an IV to stop the cramping. But after I'd been on the IV for a while, I was still feeling terrible. I was still cramping up, and I couldn't understand why.*

*Generally speaking, when a person is on an IV, it's because they're not getting enough nourishment. It's a way* to get some calories. So normal IV bags have 20% dextrose. It's sugar water.

If you're a non-diabetic, it helps you recover more quickly. But when you mainline sugar in a diabetic's veins, you dehydrate him, because his blood sugars elevate. You have to give diabetics saline IVs.

I look up and I read the IV bag, and I read that it's 20% dextrose! I started trying to rip the IV out of my arm. I told the trainers, 'You guys are a bunch of morons! What are you thinking?'

Their response was, 'Well, we never thought about it. We never had a diabetic before.'

In training camp there's usually a doctor there. They'll come in at the end of practice and ask who needs to be checked out. But they're not there through the day, so they're not constantly reminded that I have diabetes. But the training staff is.

In the excitement of having this event, the trainer assumed the doctor knew, and the doctor assumed the trainer would let him know. I didn't think the doctors were completely incompetent. They just didn't know one of the major factors concerning their patient. Or at least it didn't enter their consciousness. It was not in the normal thought process for them.

As time went by I learned that once you start cramping, it's like any of those recurring injuries, whether it's a concussion or pulled muscle; you're more susceptible to cramps once you've cramped.

*This one happened with Indianapolis. We were flying back from Miami. It was a long flight, and I don't like to fly. After a game, you're already dehydrated. On a plane they recirculate the air, so you become more dehydrated.*

*I started to have leg cramps again. Then it started turning into rib cramps, back cramps, my quads – everything started going. It feels like you're trying to break your bones or your tendons are going to pop.*

*They gave me an IV, but this time I caught it right away. I'm in the middle of these severe cramps, and I'm screaming. They thought I was screaming because of the cramps. That was part of it, but I'm also screaming because I'm telling them I can't have that IV.*

*"I can't have THAT IV," I tell them.*

*"Of course you can have an IV," they say.*

*"I can't have the IV with dextrose in it," I tell them.*

*They had one bag that was just saline solution. From that point Indianapolis always had regular saline bags on all our flights and in the training room.*

THROUGHOUT HIS career, Jay made no attempt to hide his diabetes from his teammates. Even if they ignored his occasional issues with the trainers and medical staff, and were oblivious to the all of his diabetes awareness and community service efforts, he gave them many other hard-to-miss hints.

He cut off the fingertips of the lineman's glove he wore on his left hand so he could easily and quickly test his blood sugar on the bench between offensive series. He monitored his sugar level with finger pricks many times each game. And he regularly gave himself insulin injections right at his locker.

Nonetheless, some teammates never picked up on the situation.

*With the Bears we had a guy named Jeremy Lincoln; same draft class as I, from Tennessee, a defensive back. His locker was 2-3 lockers away from me.*

*I always thought of myself as one of the hardest workers on the team; I always said that nobody could outwork me. And after a year, I knew that one of my weaknesses, no pun intended, was in the weight room. I knew I had to get bigger, stronger. I won an off-season conditioning award from the Bears for working the hardest, making the biggest improvement.*

*After being next to Jeremy for a couple years, he says to me one day: "You know, Jay, I gotta say something."*

*I say, 'Okay.'*

*He says, "You know I respect you. I think you work hard. But if you're going to take steroids, would you at least hide it, and not be so blatant in front of me?"*

*I was sitting there going, 'What?' And then I realized he had seen me take insulin injections for two years and he didn't know I was a diabetic.*

*He was so mild mannered. But he was at his wits end, as in: 'I can't take anymore. I know you're cheating. I know it's against the rules, and you're doing it right in front of me.'*

*I laughed. My attitude was, I thought everybody knew. It made sense because of all positions in football, as a lineman, I had the least contact with defensive backs. I got a big chuckle out of it, and I just used it as another opportunity to educate another soul.*

# CHAPTER 11

# ROLE MODEL

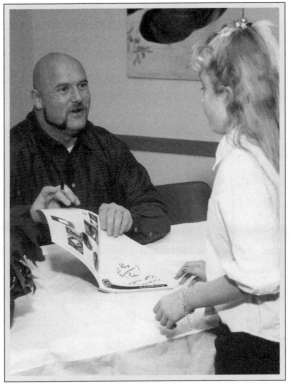

Photo courtesy of Ingher and Jay Leeuwenburg

*Lacking diabetic role models himself while*
*growing up, Jays vowed to send the message*
*to youngsters that: "You know what?*
*You can do anything you want."*

THE ROSTER of sports figures who encountered diabetes while, or after, succeeding at a highly competitive level would in itself make a Hall of Fame. Even so, some of the names would probably surprise a lot of people.

Among those who developed Type 2 (commonly known as adult onset, or non insulin-dependent, diabetes), the Famous Diabetics web site lists Wimbledon champions Arthur Ashe and Billie Jean King; baseball icon Ty Cobb, historic Jackie Robinson and Hall of Fame pitcher Catfish Hunter; heavyweight boxing champs Joe Frazier and Jersey Joe Walcott, and five-time middleweight champ Sugar Ray Robinson; Art Shell, the Hall of Fame offensive tackle who was a key part of the Oakland Raiders' Super Bowl XI and XV championships; and the legendary Adolph Rupp, who coached the University of Kentucky to four college basketball national championships and 879 victories,.

Bobby Clarke, captain of the Philadelphia Flyers' two-time Stanley Cup champions, and Ron Santo, a nine-time All-Star third baseman for the Cubs from 1960 through 1973, head the list of Type 1 (insulin-dependent) stars who preceded Jay in the national sports spotlight.

Any of them could have been role models for others dealing with the disease. Any of them could have directed their spotlight to illuminate the path for young boys and girls aspiring to emulate them as sports stars. Instead, they allowed the secret of their diabetes to remain hidden in the long shadows they cast over their sports.

Unlike world champion cyclist Lance Armstrong, who in recent years has written inspirationally about his successful battle with cancer, none chose to call attention to their disease during their careers. None chose to raise awareness and help educate the public about diabetes; None chose to send the message to millions of diabetics that they can manage their disease successfully and live a full life – whether or not they aspire to be athletes at any level.

"It was 1992 when Jay started down this path," Ingher points out. "At that point in time, there was not an athlete willing to talk about their experiences living with a disease like this. Jay was one of the first athletes to come out and say publicly that he had the disease and that, even so, he was playing football at a high level.

"People before him who had played, whether it was Ron Santo or Mike Pyle, who also played in Chicago, or any other athlete, never made it public that they had the disease during their playing careers. Jonathan Hayes was just starting to develop a relationship with the Juvenile Diabetes Foundation when Jay played with him in Kansas City, but he hadn't yet gone public.

"It was just the right opportunity, the right time. Jay opened the frontier for athletes with these diseases, and made it more comfortable for them to come out and say, 'We don't have to hide this. They don't make us any less of a competitor. They're not inhibiting my play or my teammates confidence in me as a member of the team.'

"And so you now have a whole generation of athletes that have overcome diabetes, cancer, heart disease – you name it – and they're willing to talk about it. Until Jay, they weren't."

*There were several influences, philosophies, that led me to get involved in the community and try to be a role model for people with diabetes. One is, I truly believe that while playing in the NFL, it wasn't the Bears and the McCaskeys, who owned the team, who were employing me. It was the community, the city of Chicago.*

*I felt passionately about that. From the very beginning I felt that, while obviously it was Ed McCaskey who signed my checks, this community embraced me and made me able to do this job that I loved and get very well-rewarded for it. I felt it was my obligation not only to live in the community year-round, but also to give back.*

*That was just something I came to grips with myself; it was not talked about by my parents, by my friends, by my brother. It was just something I felt was the right thing to do. That was one of the driving forces.*

*Another was how very quickly I came to grips with how you were an instant role model because you played in the NFL. You instantly have an audience and recognition and credibility. I have major issues with that now because there are a lot of less-than-desirable personalities playing in all the pro sports.*

*But it's a fact. You instantly have that audience and that voice and that credibility. Knowing that I wanted to give back to the community and knowing my voice would be heard, I asked myself how I could have the most impact given the position I was in.*

*It was a no-brainer. Growing up, I knew of no one in any sport that I could look to and even say that he or she was a diabetic, much less say that's a diabetic athlete that I wanted to emulate or that I could even seek out for advice.*

*I knew from just the mere fact of going to my normal three-month doctor visits that there were thousands upon thousands of children who were seeking answers to what I thought were just basic questions about living with and managing diabetes. And they were getting such outrageous advice that I couldn't understand. For instance, 'You can't be a cheerleader. You can't play soccer.' The message was, you can't do these things because you're a diabetic.*

*I thought it would be an injustice not to use my career and that instant credibility as a forum. So pretty early on I made it my commitment that I would send the message to youngsters that, 'You know what, you can do anything you want.'*

JAY'S BRIEF exposure to the Kansas City organization after the Chiefs drafted him also influenced his initial receptiveness to community involvement. It's almost impossible to see how being with the Chiefs, even briefly, would not make a lasting impression on anyone in this regard.

The community involvement section of the team website is called The Chiefs Way. Clicking on it in 2005, the first thing one saw was a list of community programs and activities sponsored by the football club. There were 25 of them.

The Chiefs Children's Fund, established in 1983, "provides vital support to more than 60 local youth agencies annually." The Chiefs Children's Benefit Game "is one of the largest of its kind in the NFL." The goal of Kansas City Student All-Stars is "to promote community investment and volunteerism in youth via small level grants." The Derrick Thomas Academy, "a tuition-free public charter school," opened its doors in downtown Kansas City in 2002 – "the first public elementary charter school named for an NFL hero."

The name is all you need to know to figure out what several of the programs involve. There is Out For Blood, Read Across America, Arthritis Foundation Chiefs Night, First Downs For Downs Syndrome, Kansas City's Susan B. Komen Race For The Cure, Operation Blessing Food Distribution, Gridiron Geography and Toys For Tots.

*Kansas City did an unbelievably great job of commu-
nity service and community involvement.   When you*

*signed your contract with them, you had to agree that you
would do five community outreach programs of the Chiefs'
choosing, no questions asked. That was part of your
contract. Kansas City is smaller than a lot of NFL cities.
They felt you owed it to the community.*

*I had no problem with that. When I ended up with the
Bears, part of it was me saying, 'That was a good program
in Kansas City. I do need to do something like that.' In my
mind, that was such a great initiative that somebody else
started, and I agreed with it. I needed to give back.*

*It really helped that I started becoming a more notable
player. It's a lot easier to use me as a marketing tool when
I'm actually doing good things, such as making the newspaper for my play, making the paper for my ability to stay
healthy – all the positive messages that a diabetes organization loves.*

*My attitude was, I'm helping people, and this is a by-
product of my being a good football player. It was instantly
obvious that because I played football, I instantly had credibility with the younger audience. I took very seriously
being able to use that power that was being given to me.*

*I had heard, probably after the first or second time I
had spoken to a large group of people, such comments as,
'I've said the same thing that you said for the past 10 years,
but he listened to you.' 'I've had this person as a patient for
the last six years, and they haven't done what I've told them
they need to do, but you touched something in them that has
made them change.'*

What a thrill to have a little boy come up to me and say, 'Wow, I'm going to go out for football.'

That's all the motivation I ever needed. It only takes one or two of those comments, but there were so many that I knew I had to continue.

The way I looked at it, if I reached one out of a hundred, and you give me a thousand, at least I'm reaching ten. I didn't expect that I would be changing the lives of everyone I came in contact with, but I knew from my own experience that I could at least educate parents or children that have this disease a little bit. Maybe they were just football fans who wanted an autograph, but it was okay if they learned something about diabetes, too.

For me, I was just telling my story. It's not like I was exaggerating or fabricating or doing anything more than telling my story. That was never work. It was just the right thing to do.

THE JUVENILE Diabetes Research Foundation (JDRF to most diabetics) came into existence in 1970, the year after Jay was born. It was founded by a small group of parents of children with diabetes. At first it was called just the Juvenile Diabetes Foundation.

JDRF calls itself "the largest voluntary health organization in the world raising more money to find a cure for diabetes and its complications than any other non-governmental health agency in the world." At the end of 2004, JDRF had provided more than $800 million to diabetes research worldwide.

The Foundation's mission is to find a cure for diabetes. But until that time has come, JDRF also recognizes that living with diabetes is a challenge, and so it also provides "support information for individuals and families living with insulin-dependent diabetics."

JDRF sponsors publications and public meetings, and works with schools and businesses to help them understand diabetes so they can respond more appropriately to both children and adults who are living with this disease. But the main focus is fund-raising for research.

*In football, there are always charity events. You are asked to do probably four charity events a week for the 17-week season. You can choose anything to support.*

*One of the organizations I got letters from was the Juvenile Diabetes Foundation. They just asked, "Would you be willing to give one night, have somebody pick you up in a limo, take you to a restaurant, let them pay for your dinner? All you have to do is talk to the highest bidder's son or daughter about having diabetes and playing in the NFL." That seemed so simple, so easy, that I said, 'Definitely.'*

*I happened to wind up with the son of the president of a major company in Chicago. I was expecting a little kid, but he was my age. I was 23 and he was probably 19 to 21. He was so angry at having diabetes. He hated having to check his blood sugar, and he hated having to give himself insulin injections. He was like a lot of diabetics I eventually met.*

*I think I am definitely the exception, not the rule. My emotions when I was diagnosed with diabetes, and my level of acceptance and my family support, are not the norm.*

*I've always viewed it as, 'Well, this is the hand I was dealt so I'm going to make the best of it.' It didn't matter if it was diabetes, or how tall I was, or my physical makeup. I was, and am, determined to make the best of it.*

*Unfortunately there are tenfold the people who say, "What do you mean I have to eat a certain way? What do you mean I can't continue to do this or that? What do you mean I have to get to know my body? I don't want to have to think about that.'*

*Many, many diabetics become depressed. They tend to be extremely resentful. They have the 'woe-is-me' syndrome. They wonder, 'Why did this happen to me?' They choose either to ignore their disease or not control it, or to want someone else to take care of it for them. And none of those things work.*

*There are lots of easy ways to make excuses or to refuse to accept that this is happening. And the effects to the diabetics and their families who do not deal with it are devastating,*

*I have never been hospitalized for any diabetes complication since I was diagnosed. I never missed a down of football because of diabetes. That's because I've been given some great tools that allow me to do the things I've been able to do. And they're tools that any other diabetic can use just as successfully in everyday life.*

*So many people just want it to be done with. 'If I take a shot, I'm fixed.' Well, no, you're not. You need to control this; you need to manage it, whether you're 80 or 8. One of my mottoes is: Don't let diabetes control you. Control your diabetes.*

*You don't get time off from diabetes for good behavior. You can't say, 'I've had it for 24 years, I think I'll take this month off.' You can't do that. Well, you can, but the disease is not going to be forgiving.*

CHICAGOLAND, AS the city, Cook County and five surrounding counties are collectively named, had a population approaching ten million people in the decade of the '90s. It was the nation's third largest metropolitan area.

The tracks of Chicagoland's commuter trains would stretch from Soldier Field to Omaha, and the miles of freeways linking its sprawl would continue from there all the way to Denver. Chicago itself is headquarters for ten Fortune 500 companies, among 22 in the region.

Chicagoland also is a center for the practice of medicine, as well as the teaching of the practice of medicine. Its residents are served by more than 140 hospitals, which are fed by six medical schools.

It is not particularly surprising then that Jay made more hospital visits while he played for the Bears than anywhere else in his pro career. Always, he was visiting the children. But he was trying to get through to their parents at every stop.

He would return from these visits with a variety of stories – some uplifting, some distressing – inevitably sharing them with his soul mate. It became Ingher's cause, too.

*I did a health fair at a hospital in Chicago. About 350 kids showed up. I spoke to them about my experiences, my attitudes about my personal feelings about life and diabetes. I really felt, it was one of those nights when I was extremely articulate. Everything flowed perfectly. The kids and the participants asked perfect questions. Everything went great.*

*What I remember most is the response when I was just walking out of the auditorium – not only the children but also the parents, and the impact I had on them. The parents were saying things like, 'Holy smokes! I never was giving my child the chance. I felt like I was doing the right thing by holding them back because they couldn't. But I am changing my attitude and I am going to allow my son or daughter to live their lives now.'*

*That, to me, is the biggest impact, and why I keep going back to it. You don't have enough parents who give their children enough of a chance to succeed. People are afraid of the unknown. These parents are afraid for their children. They don't know of anybody who has ever done anything as a diabetic, particularly athletically, and with the emphasis that's put on sports in our society, that's an issue. Just opening their eyes and saying, 'they can do this'* is important. *They might not succeed, but you have to give them the opportunity.*

*I visited a family in a hospital in Chicago, and I came home and told Ingher that it was truly so unfortunate that the family felt like, 'OK, we've had our three days in the hospital. We've got it all figured out. Everything's going to be great. We just bought Johnny a new Nintendo, he's starting to feel better and everything's going to be great.'*

*I remember telling Ingher, 'This family has no clue. They think that, their son got a shot of insulin, and they've changed their diet a little bit.' Their approach was, 'We're gonna do a specific meal just for him, but we're all gonna be okay.'*

*It was sad to realize how much they heard only what they wanted to hear. They did not understand. They had no clue how they were setting their son and themselves up for failure.*

*I made one hospital visit and saw two boys of almost identical age who were diagnosed within 24 hours of each other. The doctors, nurses and administration thought they were doing the right thing by putting them in a semi-private room together since they were both just starting to learn about diabetes. It was just so glaring to see the reaction of the two different sets of parents and the effect this was having on their children.*

*You had one mother who couldn't walk in the room without bursting into tears. Her son was the one who was diagnosed first, and he was still not taking his injections on his own. There was no taking control of this disease. They were still in the guilt-ridden "woe is me, how can this be happening?" stage.*

*The other family's attitude was, 'Okay, we know what's going on. We understand the things we're hearing, and we're putting our son in charge. We now know what's wrong; this is something we can live with.'*

*To have both extremes right there in the same room was phenomenal. One kid went home after only two or three days because the doctors and the nurses felt very confident in the care he was going to get at home. The parents were on the right track, and the kid was on the right track.*

*The other one spent about two weeks in the hospital. It was just amazing to see how much the differences in attitude affected the two situations.*

*I told both of them that they needed to take control of their disease, that they needed to manage it. But only one got it. He immediately asked, 'What do you do? How many units do you do when you're going to exercise?'*

CONGRESS APPROVES appropriations for the National Institute of Health, so organizations such as JDRF appear before the U.S. House of Representatives in support of funding for their particular research objectives. In Jay's third season with the Bears, he was asked by JDRF to go to Washington and tell Congress why it should increase the amount of money devoted to finding a cure for diabetes.

The messenger, however, had a different view of the right message to deliver than those who were sending him. The resulting debate with JDRF representatives reminded Ingher of the time she and Jay spoke with a producer concerning a possible movie based on Jay's life.

"When Jay got with JDRF government people and sat down to write his speech – They're very instrumental in what they want said and who you're going to say it to – there was a battle of wills. Because Jay refuses to take the victim role.

"That's the one thing about Jay; he thinks he's had a pretty darn good life and he's pretty proud about the things he's accomplished as a diabetic.

"They basically said, 'If you're not going to make these panel members cry, we're not going to get as much money.' There was quite the struggle then, between what Jay wanted to say and what they wanted him to say."

*I knew my time was very finite that I would be able to play in the NFL. Even though I had a nine-year career, that's not a very long time in the grand scheme of things. I knew I wanted to get my message out there.*

*I thought a good way to do that would be to arrange either a documentary or a movie. Ingher and I pitched the idea to a couple of people. That's when we got the response, 'It's a great story, but there's no tragedy so we can't use it.' My reaction was, 'Oh great, so I have to lose an arm or a leg or my eyesight, and then you'll be interested.'*

*JDRF wanted very strongly for me to say that I was a person afflicted with this horrible, terrible, incurable disease, and my life has been ruined by it. I told them I wasn't comfortable saying that.*

*I said, 'I'm a diabetic.' You would have thought I called them a dirty word. Their reaction was, 'You CANNOT say THAT!' And I said, 'Why not?'*

*They basically told me JDRF is not a proponent of labeling diabetics as diabetics, because it's a disease. You have a "disease." You are not "a diabetic."*

*I was so ticked. Not one of these people telling me this had the disease themselves. I said, 'Hello. I'm a diabetic. I'm a male. It's who I am. I'm okay with that.' It was as if they were saying, 'If you brand yourself a diabetic, you're less of a person.' My feeling was, 'No. The only reason you would think that is that you think that way."*

*Some people tried to turn it into, 'Either you want to find a cure or you don't.' I'd tell them, of course I want to find a cure. Their answer was, 'Well then, all your efforts and fund-raising should go toward medical research.' Their feeling was, if they use the money on education and on how to have a lifestyle that can be healthy now, they're taking money away from medical research.*

*That might be right up to a point. But as a diabetic living with this disease, I'm not willing to mortgage my future by saying, 'Okay, fine, I'm going to put all my efforts and energy into that.'*

*I've been taking four shots a day for more than 20*

*years. The frustrating thing is, I was told when I was diagnosed, 'There'll be a cure within ten years.' Today, newly diagnosed diabetics are being told, 'There'll be a cure in ten years. I'm going to do everything I can to make that become a reality. But meanwhile I need to be living a healthy life, to make myself able to be productive until that time comes.*

*I heard what they said, and they heard what I said. They wanted me to say I have Type 1 Diabetes, rather than saying I am a diabetic. I relinquished on that point, but I wasn't going to go in there with a sob story.*

*My message to Congress was, 'Look at me. The reason I'm successful is because of the research you have invested in.' It was right after Humalog, a faster-acting insulin, became available. Mine was a really positive message: 'I'm succeeding because the technology and research you've invested in is bringing results. What we're saying is, the results can be even bigger if there's more money going into it. And ultimately a cure, so we don't have these sob stories.'*

*I was so tired of being constantly told, basically, that it's okay to be a victim, that it's okay to feel like you can't do this because you have this horrible, terrible disease that's incurable. A large portion of the population takes on what I'll call the victim role. Their response would be, 'It's not a choice we have; it's because of this devastating disease.' To which I say, 'Baloney.'*

*That's my mission: To say you do have a choice. Is it always going to be easy? Heck no. Are you going to have to work hard? Absolutely. Should you take it lying down* and not be an active participant? No way.

I would say this whether I had diabetes or not. But I've been in the spotlight because of my profession. I feel it's my duty to educate people that it's not helpless and hopeless.

My feeling is there are plenty of successful programs for plenty of problems – substance abuse or alcoholism, for examples. You talk about all these programs that you go to, or through, and in all of them you accept responsibility and take an active role in your life. They're successful because they acknowledge, 'Hey, I have "this",' whatever "this" is.

JDRF didn't ask me back because, truly, they want to play on the sentimental. They want to bring in a kid who's crying and says he's dying, and says, 'If you give me more money I won't die, but if you won't give me more money through National Institute of Health spending, then you will have killed me.

Dr. Wolff taught me, and my parents raised me with the belief, that you are all about this disease and how it's going to affect you, and that you have control over it. That's the way you can live successfully with it until there's a cure.

CHAPTER 12

# JAY'S CORNER

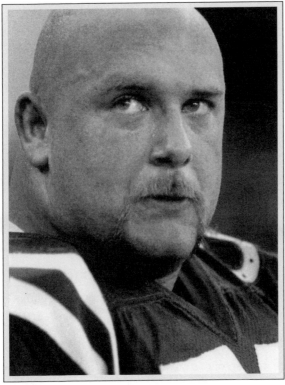

Photo courtesy of Indianapolis Colts Football Club

*"Through your generosity," wrote a school nurse,*
*"I saw some special, caring young people see*
*the Colts game and share their excitement with you.*
*You have touched their lives."*

THE HEADLINE on the front page of the *Rocky Mountain News* read, **"New Deal Brings Free Agency, Salary Cap To NFL."** The date was January 7, 1993, a Thursday.

"Working under a judge's deadline, the NFL and its players agreed Wednesday on a seven-year contract that brings unrestricted free agency and a salary cap to professional football," the story distributed by The Associated Press began.

"The contract, which runs through 1999, includes a free-agency plan that allows players with more than five NFL seasons' experience to become unrestricted free agents. If player costs reach 67% of designated NFL gross revenues, a salary cap goes into effect and players can become free agents after four years.

"The agreement is the first since 1987, when players struck for 24 days, then went back to work without a contract."

Jay was entering his second year in the league when the news broke. Dave Wannstedt would not be named head coach of the Bears for 12 more days. Jay's first start of his career was still eight months away.

Nevertheless, it was a life-changing day for Jay, one that would pay off handsomely just a few years later. Right after he completed his fourth season, in fact.

Published with the story was a summary of the most significant provisions of the new contract. Two, in particular, regarding exceptions to free agency and a change in the college draft, would influence not only Jay's professional career but also his future financial security.

"Each team will be able to exempt one "franchise" player from free agency for the duration of his career if he is offered a contract at the average of at least the top five players at his position," wrote Associated Press. "In 1993 each team will be able to use the right of first refusal on two of its free agents if they are offered a contract at the average of at least the top 10 players at their positions. In 1994 every club will have one right of first refusal under the same conditions as '93.

"The college draft will be reduced to seven rounds, plus an extra round for teams that lose free agents."

*My class was the very first draft class that was able to be unrestricted free agents after four years in the league. If you weren't under contract you could go shop yourself to any team in the league. That's when player salaries started taking off. It was a whole new world for the owners, the GMs and the players.*

*When I was drafted, I wanted to sign a one-year*

contract because I was confident I'd be playing my first year. I thought I could get a better deal after I showed what I could do. But the minimum contract you could sign was two years, so I signed a two-year contract. So my contract was up in two years. But you have to have four years to be a free agent, so I signed a one-year deal my third year.

After the third year you were called a restricted free agent. That meant, as the title suggests, the team could put a restriction on you. You could go out and get an offer from another team, but that other team had to let the club you were under contract with match the offer, and they had to give up a draft pick equal to the round you were drafted in if you wound up signing with them.

Since they had reduced the draft to seven rounds and I was drafted in the ninth round, the Bears weren't going to get any draft choice compensation if another team signed me. But there was a catch to the restricted free agent, a dollar amount. The Bears tendered me a $700,000 offer, so if another team wanted to match that, they'd have to give up first-round draft choice to the Bears.

This is where I started having difficulty with Ted Phillips. He was chief financial officer and did all the contracts when I was there. He later became president of the Bears.

My contract negotiation approach through my agent was really pretty simple: If you think I'm good enough to put a first round draft restriction on me, then sign me to a long-term deal so we don't have to go through this when I

*become an unrestricted free agent. I was willing and want-*
*ing to sign a long-term contract with the Bears.*

*Ted told me, "Nobody's going to want you. You're not*
*going to play that much. If you do, you're not going to*
*make that much money."*

*This was very typical George Halas. I had heard*
*stories that Halas would literally show you three hours of*
*your worst plays from practice and games, then offer you're*
*a horrible contract and make you feel like you should be*
*begging to play for the team. So this was deeply entrenched:*
*to downgrade the ability of your player and try to pay him*
*less. I believe Ted was in that tradition.*

*It was then, when I didn't like those negotiation*
*tactics, that I told him it would be extremely difficult for me*
*to come back as a free agent and sign a contract with the*
*Bears if they didn't even attempt to negotiate with me now.*
*And as an unrestricted free agent I would demand a larger*
*salary. He said, "We're willing to risk it."*

COMING OFF a season in which they surprised the NFL by not
only making the playoffs but also winning that first-round game
over the Vikings before getting clobbered 45-10 by eventual
Super Bowl XXIX champion San Francisco, the Bears went into
the 1995 season believing they were contenders in their division.
They had bolstered the weakest part of their attack, their
running game, by drafting the Heisman Trophy winner, Rashaan
Salaam, from Jay's alma mater, and everything else was pretty

much intact from the year before.

The most significant change occurred not on the field, but in the front office. General manager Bill Tobin, the man who spotted Jay on the waiver wire as Kansas City tried to sneak him through back in the summer of '92, was fired, only to be hired a short time later by the Indianapolis Colts.

An undefeated October left the Bears with a 6-2 record and thoughts of home field advantage in the playoffs halfway through the schedule. But the second verse was not the same as the first. They lost five of their next six.

Chicago needed a victory over Eastern Division champion Philadelphia in the final game of the season just to match the previous season's 9-7 record. If favored San Francisco could beat Atlanta, that 9-7 would qualify for the post-season.

Salaam ran for 1,074 yards, breaking the 61-year-old club record for yards rushing by a rookie. But there was no post-season for him and Jay. The Falcons rallied and upset the 49ers, earning the last playoff spot themselves. The season-ending victory over the Eagles was Jay's last game as a member of the Chicago Bears.


*I ended up signing a contract with Bill Tobin soon after the free agency signing period began. It was the third year in a row I started every game. I was an alternate to the Pro Bowl. And at the time, Indianapolis seemed the most interested, particularly monetarily. They wanted to move very quickly.*

*I was flown down for a visit; Bill Tobin offered me a contract and told me I had one hour to make a decision. That's the way he worked. He didn't want me to shop my offer.*

*Having gone through a physical with two other centers they brought in at the same time, I knew he meant it. He said if you don't want this offer, I'm prepared to make this offer to the guy right behind you.*

*He was offering me great money and a long-term contract, $6.3 million for four years. That included a signing bonus – $1.5 million to sign. It was life-changing. It is, still.*

*Tobin understood it was a big risk for me. If I didn't take that offer, I might not get an offer like it later from anyone else. No one else had put money on the table at that point.*

*Only the bonus was guaranteed; I had to be on the team to get the rest. My first year was worth a million dollars. My next year I got one-point-one, then I made one-point-two. The last year I was supposed to make $1.5 million.*

*It made me the highest paid center in the league at that time. Ted Phillips came out in the Chicago papers and said he offered me the same contract and I had rejected it, which was an outright lie.*

*You'll never win an argument in the paper. The fans and the media are mad at you because you're leaving their town. They say good riddance to you. I never even responded to what Phillips had said.*

THE BANNER proclaiming "Jay's Corner" went up in a corner section of seats in the RCA Dome at the start of the 1997 season. In the beginning, there were 30 seats for every Colts home game, paid for entirely by Jay and Ingher. A year later it grew to 150 seats when Eli Lilly & Company and Roche Diagnostics, Indianapolis-based companies on which diabetics everywhere have come to rely, partnered with Jay and Ingher.

Children with Type 1 diabetes from all over Indiana and their families were invited to request tickets. Winners chosen by lottery drawing received four tickets for seats in Jay's Corner. They were encouraged to use one of the tickets to bring a member of their "diabetes team" as a guest, perhaps a dietician, a teacher or the school nurse.

The idea was to enable children and their support system to see Jay "at work" – accomplishing what most children with diabetes think they can only dream of accomplishing. Along with seeing what for most was their first NFL game, winners of the ticket lottery also got to meet Jay in person.

The "Thank You" notes that followed document the impact of this extraordinary effort.

"Our daughter is Lauren," began the parents of visitor to Jay's Corner. "She is 8 and was diagnosed at age 5. What a thrill to see her expression upon entering the RCA Dome and seeing the Colts for the first time. She talks about Jay all the time and has his poster hanging in her bedroom. You are such an inspiration to her and so many other kids with diabetes."

A school nurse wrote: "Through your generosity, I saw some special, caring young people have the opportunity to see the Colts game and to share their excitement with you. Five young men who spelled out "Go Jay" on their abdomens, and a little blonde-haired girl who invited me to attend with her and her family, were truly excited. You have touched their lives."

*I arranged a place where I would meet with every family. I would spend sometimes three hours after the game talking with them. And there could be 100 to 150 people hanging out. I just told them to meet me by the stadium door, and we'd just hang out.*

*Ingher would always have a big spread there, like a deli sandwich and a big cooler of diet soda. It was usually just for me because I'd be starving, and everybody felt liked they'd be imposing. But, you know, I'd always have a couple of regular Cokes on hand, too, in case somebody got low.*

*I really wanted to make sure that they understood that I thought it was important that they see a diabetic in action. You could hear it and watch it on TV, but I thought it was really something special to be able to go to the game and see somebody that has the same disease as you did. For the most part you have been told you can't go do this, and then you see this guy doing it with your eyes.*

*And not only that. Questions come up and it's a more informal setting so they feel they can ask you questions.*

COLTS FANS were still reliving the agonizing sight of the potential game-winning touchdown pass barely eluding receiver Aaron Bailey in the end zone on the final play of the AFC Championship game when Jay accepted Bill Tobin's lucrative offer. Because the Colts had come that close to going to the Super Bowl, optimism for the next season tempered the disappointment.

Indy had been to the playoffs two seasons in a row, and had upset top-seeded Kansas City the week before losing to Pittsburgh. That one was triumph under the harshest conditions imaginable: in minus-9 wind chill and at Arrowhead Stadium, widely acknowledged as the loudest, least hospitable place for a visiting team in the NFL.

The Colts offense was loaded with a future Hall of Fame running back, Marshall Faulk; a new threat in rookie wide receiver Marvin Harrison, who would draw coverage away from veteran Sean Dawkins; and a proven quarterback, Jay's former Bears teammate, Jim Harbaugh.

The up-and-coming team Jay thought he had joined, though, turned out to be mostly an illusion. As good as the offense was, it was outscored each of the next three seasons. The defense allowed 401 points in '97 and an unimaginable 444 in '98.

Instead of stability, Jay was battered by change, beginning even before he donned the helmet with the horseshoe on it for the first time. He endured the worst seasons of his football career – at any level – and wound up leaving the Colts before collecting everything his long-term contract had promised.

*You sign a great contract. Go to a team that's up and coming. Everything looks great. I really felt like we were going someplace.*

*We went 9-7, and lost to Pittsburgh in the first round of the playoffs. The next season we went 3-13. Then they draft Peyton Manning. I'm now center in Peyton Manning's rookie year. We go 3-13 again. It happened that fast.*

*When I signed my free agent contract, Ted Marchibroda was the coach. By the time I got down there, he was gone and Lindy Infante was the coach. Making the playoffs that first year was the last success we had.*

*The most memorable part of that game for me didn't really have anything to do with the final score. I was playing guard and Kirk Loudermilk was the center. Jim Harbaugh was our quarterback.*

*We were playing in Three Rivers Stadium, and it was loud. Kirk snapped the ball early, and our left tackle never made it out of his stance. Chad Brown came off the corner and just annihilated Harbaugh, just killed him.*

*We're in the huddle, and Jim starts talking. But nobody can understand him. We said, 'What the heck are you saying?'*

*He mumbles, 'Hold on,' and he pulls his two front teeth out of his mouth. He's got blood streaming out of his mouth, and he couldn't enunciate the words. He'd lost his teeth!*

*He took his teeth, and he put them in his sock. I remember looking at him and thinking, 'That's disgusting.' You don't usually have that sort of feeling in the middle of a playoff game, but that was just gross.*

*Jim is one of the toughest guys I've ever known. He didn't miss a play. He couldn't put his mouthpiece in because his mouth was so swollen, so he got one for his bottom teeth. We lost 42-14.*

*We went 3-13 the next season, and Lindy got fired. Then they brought in Jim Mora. That was Peyton Manning's rookie year. We went 3-13 again.*

MANY NFL teams hold their pre-season training camps on college campuses. For years the Cincinnati Bengals went to Wilmington College, 50 miles north; the Denver Broncos set up at the University of Northern Colorado, also about 50 miles up the road. This custom had something to do with isolating the players so they could focus of football, and building camaraderie and bonding as a team by sharing dorm rooms.

While Jay was with the Colts, they settled on Terre Haute and the campus of Rose-Hulman Institute of Technology as their summertime home away from home. Terre Haute shares the approximate longitude of Chicago and is only slightly above the latitude of St. Louis, which is to say it's suffocatingly humid there, too.

It doesn't help that the Wabash River curves through Terre Haute on its way to joining up first with the Ohio River on the edge of Western Kentucky and then the mighty Mississippi at Cairo, just a little farther south. Significant rivers contribute to the discomfort of summer in places like Terre Haute.

Colts summer camp there was not much fun under any

circumstances. Under a new head coach looking to establish his
brand of tough football, it was even worse.

*Indiana summers were just brutal: no breeze, 90-plus
temperature and humidity. You'd listen on the radio, and
they would give cattle warnings, that you needed to watch
your livestock so they didn't get overheated in the fields.*

*But we would practice for two-plus hours in that heat.
We'd say to the coaches, 'You wouldn't let your cow out
there in this stuff, but you definitely let us practice.'*

*There was a day during Mora's first camp when he
just brutalized us. We were out there well over three hours.*

*The practice fields at Rose-Hulman were sunken, so
you're in this valley. We had to walk up a hill to go to the
dining hall. I was walking up the stairs, up the hill, and I
started cramping in my hamstrings. I thought, 'Uh-oh, I
don't think I'm going to make it.'*

*I barely made it back to the training room before I had
the worst full body cramps I've ever had. When I got there,
there were 26 players in the training room with full body
cramps! One of my fellow linemen was is such bad shape
he had to be taken to the hospital. They had to give him not
only the intravenous fluids – I believe he had six bags of IV
– but they also had to give him two shots of valium just to
calm him down.*

*That's how insane it was. You'd wake up and feel like
every muscle in your body has been beaten with a baseball*

*bat because it had been cramped so tight. You felt like you were in a car wreck, not only because of the collisions in practice but because every muscle has been cramped.*

*My quads were cramped so tight, it felt like my kneecap was going to break because my leg was going to hyperextend. I remember screaming, asking a guy to sit on my foot with my leg over a bucket to try to get it to bend because it hurt so bad.*

*There was another guy who was even worse. He was a new guy on the team, a defensive back. The one place where there was shade was a mulch path. The DB after every play would jog over and rest in that one spot of shade. It turned out he was allergic to tree bark. He started producing all this mucous. He almost died.*

*You saw some crazy things happen in that camp. We had practice the next day.*

READING ONLY the summary of the 1998 season in the Colts Media Guide, no one would ever guess Indianapolis won only three games and was outscored by 134 points.

> (11/1) QB Peyton Manning set a club rookie record with a TD pass in his fifth straight game, while Faulk tied a club record (shared with RBs Lenny Moore and Lydell Mitchell) with his fifth consecutive 1,000+ yards/scrimmage season.

> (11/29) Colts return to Baltimore marked by Manning's club rookie record third 300+ game (27-42-357), Faulk's

club record 267 yards/scrimmage (17-192, 1 TD rushing/ 7-75, 1 receiving) and 9-153, 1 TD receiving effort by WR-Torrance Small.

(12/6) Manning broke the 50-year old NFL rookie mark (held by QB-Charlie Conerly, NYG, 1948) with a TD pass in a 10th straight game.

(12/13) Manning ended game vs. Cincinnati with 286-502-3,179 totals to set NFL rookie records for completions (274, Mirer, Sea.), attempts (486, Mirer, Sea.) and TDs (22, Conerly, NYG). He set an NFL rookie record with his fourth 3 TD game.

(12/20) Manning set NFL rookie record and tied club seasonal record (QB-John Unitas, 1960, 1963) with fourth 300+ game. He ended game at Seattle with 309 seasonal completions, 3,514 yards and scoring tosses in 14 different games, surpassing prior respective records of QBs-Jeff George (292, 1991), Unitas (3,481, 1963) and Earl Morrall (13, 1968).

*It was a difficult year, not only because we played so poorly, but also because it wasn't fun. Peyton threw 28 interceptions. I know because I had to cover them all. It was dreadful.*

*I had gotten spoiled, coming from the Bears who made it to the playoffs, and going to the Colts and the first year they're in the playoffs. Two straight 3-13 seasons – to win six games in two seasons – was hard going.*

*In the small world that it is, Howard Mudd was my offensive line coach in Indianapolis. I'd been cut only once in the NFL, slash, traded to Chicago from Kansas City, and Howard Mudd was my line coach then. So as soon as Jim Mora was hired by the Colts and he named Howard the offensive line coach, I knew my days were numbered. Certain coaches don't like certain personalities and players.*

*In the off-season they traded Marshall Faulk to St. Louis, and drafted Edgerrin James from Miami. With Peyton and Marvin Harrison already there, they were thinking they were a year or two away. They were building for the future, and I was a veteran they didn't feel was worth as much money as my contract was going to be.*

*I felt I had a lot of factors moving against me. I had age against me because they were looking three years down the road. In three more years I would have been that much more expensive and I would have been that much older. And Bill Tobin was gone, and he was the one, as general manager, who was in my corner.*

*I was going into the last year of my contract. So they chose not to bring me back so they wouldn't have to pay me that money. I ended up getting only three years of my deal.*

*I knew they had a very young team, they were rebuilding and I was too expensive. I asked them to release me before training camp so I could go to another training camp. They wouldn't release me because I was their insurance policy in case anybody got hurt.*

*I was antsy. I wanted to get out of there because I expected to play, so I needed to get somewhere and learn the offense. They wound up releasing me a week before the season!*

*I really felt I was wronged, and I was an angry man. I felt I still had a lot of football left in me. I felt I was still a very good football player.*

*The timing stunk. What happens is that teams fall in love with the players who are there. It's sort of a self-fulfilling prophecy that if you see this guy in camp and you see his strengths and weaknesses, and you mold your offense around that, it's very difficult for coaches to say, 'Wait a minute, how would a Jay Leeuwenburg fit it?'*

*But small worlds are small worlds. Bill Tobin's son, Duke, was second in command for pro scouting for the Bengals. He actually had been a college teammate of mine, too.*

*And the defensive line coach was Tim Krumrie. I had played against him. He remembered me as a player, remembered playing against me, and remembered me as a good player. So I had two people on the staff, who both had high regard for me. That helped.*

*I signed with Cincinnati.*

THE DECISION to cut Jay created a public relations problem the Colts either underestimated or didn't anticipate, even though they should have. He had started 37 straight games, and Jay's

Corner had grown in popularity.

"Prior to the start of training camp, back in May and in early June," Mora told the media, "we brought Jay in and told him that we were going to rotate him with Larry Moore and Waverly Jackson. We told him that we felt like we had some good young offensive linemen here that we wanted to take a look at.

"We told Jay that he would have the chance to compete for a starting job. But as camp progressed, we decided that we wanted to go with Larry at center and Waverly at guard. We thought that they had played well enough through training camp to have the opportunity to start for us."

Mora's quotes appeared in an Associated Press story dated August 31, 1999. The invitation to enter the Jay's Corner lottery for the coming season had gone out just a few weeks before.

The first home game that year was September 12. The awkward letter from the Colts to families across Indiana was dated September 21.


TO WHOM IT MAY CONCERN:


Jay and Ingher Leeuwenburg work closely with the Juvenile Diabetes Foundation, Eli Lilly & Company and Roche Diagnostics in educating communities locally and nationally concerning diabetes. Such involvement in the community gives the Leeuwenburg's satisfaction knowing they are touching lives and educating the public with their programs.

One such program is "Jay's Corner." "Jay's Corner" (a ticket bloc of 150 tickets) was established in Indianapolis in 1997 to provide families and children effected with the same disease as Jay an opportunity to see a professional football player perform at a professional level in a National Football League game. Tickets for "Jay's Corner" are distributed through a lottery system.

"Jay's corner" was developed to include the NFL organization Jay is currently playing for. **"Jay's Corner" will not be in place in Indianapolis this year** unfortunately, due to Jay's transition to the Cincinnati Bengals.

The partnership between Eli Lilly & Company, Roche Diagnostics and the Leeuwenburgs appreciates your support and apologizes for any inconvenience this transition has caused.

CHAPTER 13

# LIFE-SIZE

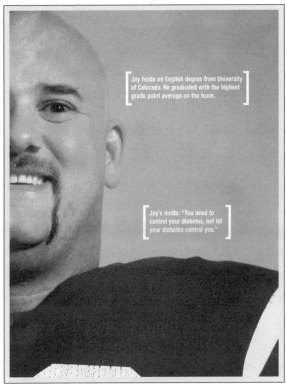

Poster reproduced courtesy of Roche Diagnostics

*"We want kids with juvenile diabetes to be like
every other kid and fit in," Jay said when his
life-size poster won a national award.
"This poster is a great way to make that happen."*

COLONEL ELI Lilly, a pharmacist by trade who became an officer in the Union Army during the Civil War, returned to central Indiana after Appomattox, acquired a small laboratory and founded Eli Lilly & Co. in 1876. Twenty years later Fritz Hoffmann, then newly married to Adele La Roche, started a small pharmaceutical specialties company in Basel, Switzerland.

Though continents and worlds apart, Col. Lilly and Dr. Hoffmann shared a similar vision: develop and produce medicines for the masses.

Lilly's idea to coat pills with gelatin helped put his company on the medical map before the turn of the century. And in 1923, under son Josiah's leadership, Lilly & Co. capitalized on the development of insulin at the University of Toronto in 1919 and became the first company to successfully mass produce the life-saving replacement for the hormone diabetics are missing.

Hoffman's single laboratory, meanwhile, grew into Roche

Holding Ltd., named for his wife. At first the company focused on pharmaceuticals, but a desire for innovation led to adding the diagnostic side of medical practice.

Both companies prospered spectacularly until, a century later, Eli Lilly & Company had more than 30,000 employees working in 170 countries, and Roche employed double that in 150 countries.

The two were credited with hundreds of new drugs, improved drugs, and other medical advancements. Among them were the Accu-Chek line of blood monitors and insulin pumps, produced by the Roche Diagnostics division; Humulin, the first genetically engineered insulin, introduced by Lilly in 1983, and its cousin Humalog, a more flexible synthetic insulin product that Lilly brought to the American market in 1996.

The two healthcare giants made Indianapolis the ideal place for a diabetic professional athlete who wanted to call attention to his disease rather than hide it.

*Eli Lilly's world headquarters is in Indianapolis. They make all the insulin I've ever used, that helps keep me alive. And Roche Diagnostics has their North American headquarters in Indianapolis. They make a blood monitoring system that is a tool that helps me monitor how much sugar is in my blood. They have done a great job of advancing technology to that check more accurate and a lot quicker.*

*When I got to Indianapolis, I was at the peak of my career. I had just made alternate to the Pro Bowl. I had just signed the biggest contract for a center at the time. It lasted only about a week, but after that I was one of the top five paid centers in the league.*

*I was going into my fifth year, so I knew I'd already passed the life expectancy of a pro football player. Players didn't make it, on average, past their third year. So I understood the power of being a celebrity, but also how fragile it was. I felt I had to strike while the iron was hot.*

*Ingher and I had been so involved in trying to raise awareness of diabetes, and we were becoming more involved. We said there has got to be some way we can put these things together.*

*It made no sense for the one NFL player who has diabetes, who's playing in this city, not to do something with Lilly and Roche. It would be stupid o all three of us. The increase in my profile as a player, and the fact that we really felt like we had a great message that needed to get out there – why in the world wouldn't these companies want to be part of this?*

*It makes sense, but it wasn't that easy. Part of the difficulty was that I didn't have an agent and didn't go to them saying, 'Here's the idea and it will cost you $20,000, but this is the proposal and here's what you'll get out of it.*

*I made zero money on these things, which still to this day is fine. It's never ever been my impetus. But in the crazy way the business world works, there may have been a different push or focus had I gone in there and convinced Lilly or Roche that they could make a bundle of money rather than just sending a good message.*

*Obviously it all ended up working out. At least 90%*
*of the credit goes to Ingher. She really, really worked hard*
*to make it happen. I would have gotten too frustrated and*
*said the heck with the whole thing. But she wouldn't let me.*

GOOD IDEAS don't always originate in a single, brilliant mind
with more creativity and imagination than anyone else's. Often
they are the sum of several good thoughts, added and mixed and
modified as the brainstorming feeds on itself.

At the end of such a session, no one can remember who
actually suggested whatever it is that suddenly has everyone
nodding excitedly. That's because no one remembers just how
the final plan was hatched. It just happened.

The Jay Leeuwenburg life-size motivational/educational
diabetes poster for kids, in fact, came about just that way, according to Ingher.

"When we were in Chicago and Jay was on the JDF Board,"
she explains, "one of the other board members worked at the
Edelman Agency. Edelman is one of the top public relations
firms in the country. She kept saying, 'You know what, this is a
great thing. We need to get Jay out there. We need to be using
him in more of this (JDF promotion).'

"Then Jay signed with the Colts. It was like hand-delivering
Eli Lilly and Roche Diagnostics the dream PR machine at the very
time the Food and Drug Administration started allowing pharmaceutical companies to advertise their products. Our friend from

Chicago said, 'Okay, I'll start making some calls for you.' "

This was years before Dan Reeves, who played and coached in Super Bowls during his long NFL career, began extolling the virtues of a certain cholesterol management drug in national television commercials. And before Mike Ditka and baseball star Rafael Palmeiro were regularly seen during "breaks in the action" pitching male sex medications on sports telecasts.

"In the early 90s," Ingher reminds, "this was not an approach pharmaceutical companies took. They did not do PR. They did not pursue advertising. That has all been a new wave that started when the FDA opened them up to advertising. Jay was that first athlete.

"Maybe because advertising was so new for pharmaceutical companies at that time, it was like pulling teeth. You would have thought they would have been ready for this. We ended up setting up a lot of programs and then going back to Lilly and Roche and saying, 'We want you to be supportive of these, then we'll do this for you.' Instead of paying Jay to be their spokesman, they bought season tickets for Jay's Corner and sponsored the poster.

"That's how the poster came about. We had set up the ticket block for Jay's Corner. But our vision was bigger. We wanted to buy more tickets. We wanted to set up more services for these kids."

Eventually, Jay and Ingher began meeting with representatives of Roche, Lilly and the Majestic Group, an Indianapolis marketing firm. They ruled out any kind of book because Roche had previously done one. They considered a video and some other ideas, but settled on the poster because Roche wanted to promote their involvement in diabetes camps.

"From the get-go, the poster was a cumulative thing," Ingher recalls. "The poster wasn't necessarily an agenda item when we all walked into that first meeting. By the end of the meeting, when we said this is what we want to offer to these kids, the poster came up as the best option. It was a collaborative effort on how we could get to these kids."

*When we were in the negotiation part with Eli Lilly and Roche about the poster, there was a young man out of Ohio State. He played cornerback, and he was diabetic and highly drafted, I think in the second round.*

*He ended up in training camp going into an insulin coma. Part of me thought, 'Oh my goodness.' You feel for the kid, but at the same time, I felt like so much of my work had just instantly gotten flushed down the toilet. Any other stereotype was instantly, 'Well . . . SEE'*

*I tend to be tough on other diabetics. It takes a lot of work. It takes an extreme amount of self-discipline. And it also takes a great self-knowledge of your body. You have to condition yourself.*

*And you're put in incredibly stressful situations, particularly physically and mentally, in the NFL. I don't think very many people can handle it, diabetic or not. For as much good as I've done, it's easy for people to say, 'He's the exception.'*

*One of the reasons I didn't get hurt in the NFL is because I had a purpose in my training. I was fortunate enough to have someone in my life in the sports training field, and I trained differently enough. Ingher and I talked a lot about the hamstring-quad ratio when we were working out.*

*Ingher had seen enough people with blown-out knees. Generally speaking, football players' quads are about twice as strong as their hamstrings. The first thing you do when you recover from a knee injury is make that closer to 1-to-1. The obvious question is, why is it that you have to blow your knee out before you do that? So I made it a specific emphasis to strengthen my hamstrings.*

*The other thing was that my awareness of the game made me better able to anticipate some of those freak situations. Having said that, how much did that help, maybe ten percent? But that ten percent might have been the difference between my having an ankle that needed to be cleaned up and my having total knee reconstruction. I wore knee braces every game I ever played.*

*I feel like, yes, there are some fortunate circumstances, but I also feel like there are some very specific things I did with my football career, my training and my diabetes. If you know maintaining good blood sugar level decreases your chances of complications, why not do it? Why wait?*

*I was very, very conscious of the position I put myself in because I put myself up as a role model. I was very aware that if those 150 kids are at a Colts game and all of a sudden it's, 'Oh, Jay just passed out!' – I mean, What kind of*

*message is Yes I Can, Yes You Can? I'm not trying to say*
*I'm perfect in any way, shape or form. But there's a little*
*extra responsibility there.*

*You don't get time off from diabetes for good behavior.*
*This is something you have to deal with every minute of*
*your life.*

*As I've said before, I've never been hospitalized and I*
*never missed a down of football because of diabetic compli-*
*cations, period. The football I missed was because of that*
*foot infection, not because I had diabetes. I never missed a*
*practice in college, never missed a practice in the pros. I*
*never missed a start because of diabetic complications; I*
*never pulled myself out of a game, and I never passed out.*

*Not that it's a horrible thing to have any of these*
*things happen, but I think it's a little extra responsibility*
*that helps me make sure that I maintain and manage my*
*diabetes, maybe better than I otherwise would have.*

THE U.S. FOOD and Drug Administration's Center for Drug
Evaluation and Research does much more than just review the
safety and effectiveness of new medicines before approving
them for sale to the public. The Division of Drug Marketing,
Advertising and Communications regulates the messages
consumers receive about drug products, from labeling and pack-
aging to marketing and public service announcements.

Two excerpts from the Division's Frequently Asked
Questions (FAQ) section concerning Consumer-Directed

Advertisements capture the constraints and controls under which Jay's poster was produced.

Question: What is a reminder advertisement?

Answer: Under 202.1(e)(2)(i), reminder advertisements "call attention to the name of the drug product but do not include indications or dosage recommendations for use of the drug product . . . and, optionally, information . . . containing no representation or suggestion relating to the advertised drug product." Reminder advertisements cannot make a representation about the product or suggest a use for the product.

Question: Does FDA limit the amount of money that can be spent on reminder advertisements or reminder labeling pieces or regulate the types of objects (such as pens, cups, calendars etc.) that can be used as reminder advertisements or reminder labeling pieces?

Answer: FDA regulations do not limit how much money companies may spend on reminder advertisements or labeling pieces, nor do the regulations limit the types of objects that can be used. The regulations, however, limit the type of information that can be presented in reminder advertisements and labeling pieces, and not just written information, but information that may be portrayed through graphics, design or some other visual representation.

"The poster is as close as you can get to preserving Jay's personality in a litigious environment," Ingher almost sighs with resignation. "Everything on that poster had to be approved by both Eli Lilly's attorneys, Roche's attorneys and the FDA.

"There are no dosages mentioned. He couldn't say, 'I take ten units in the morning' – that type of thing. The calorie count was very strife-ridden, and when he talks about his diet, because you don't want a teenage boy thinking he can eat like that.

"If it comes through and anyone who knows Jay senses any of the person he is, we did a great job. Because there were so many things we could not use."

*When we were deciding what to put on the poster, we really liked the life-size idea. Part of that was having the growth chart, then contrasting my diabetic regimen to other diabetics, letting them realize what I had to go through*

*We also wanted to give them some information – who is this guy Jay? 'I like this and I do this, but I'm really a normal every-day kind of guy.'*

THE POSTER is big enough to fill a doorway. It features a full-height photo of Jay in his No. 58 uniform, holding his helmet in his right hand and gripping a football in his left. The uniform is Colts blue, but by design, neither the team name nor the trademark horse-shoe insignia is anywhere to be seen. The Indianapolis Colts Football Club did not support the poster in any way.

From head to toe, the bright orange background is peppered with information about Jay and how he manages his diabetes. Up the left side is a 6-foot 3-inch ruler so that the giant poster can double as a growth chart.

Jay's autograph and the Yes I Can! Yes You Can! logo occupy a space almost a foot in diameter near the top of the poster. Within its 18 square feet are a dozen tidbits and three sections called Jay's Stats, Jay's Routine and Jay's Diet.

Jay's Stats highlights Jay's personal and family history, his involvement in JDF, his college football career, and some distinctions during his NFL seasons. Among the latter: "Behind Jay, Chicago led the NFL in allowing the fewest quarterback sacks (15) in 1995," and "Started every game in 1997 season, helping Marshall Faulk rush for 1,054 yards and 7 touchdowns," and "Has started at center, right guard, left guard, right tackle and left tackle."

The tidbits begin around Jay's hairless head and smiling, Fu Manchu-ed face:

Jay shaves his head twice a week and has
been doing so for five years. (He likes the look.)

Jay holds an English degree from University
of Colorado. He graduated with the highest
grade point average on the team.

Jay's fierce determination and positive
attitude serve him on the field – and off.

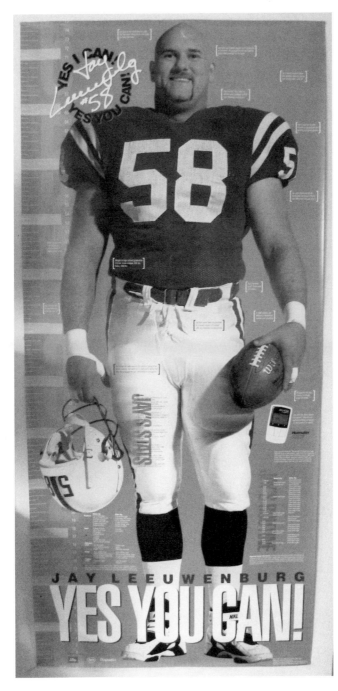

Poster reproduced courtesy of Roche Diagnostics

Jay's motto: "You need to control your
diabetes, not let your diabetes control you."

\* \* \* \* \*

From Jay's shoulders to his waist are "inside" notes every
young fan would want to know:

Jay's hobbies include traveling,
racquetball and playing computer games.

Jay once lifted two 90-lb dumbbells 40 times!
(That's like lifting two 10-year-olds!)

Jay's favorite food?
Chocolate ice cream.

Weight at high school graduation: 220 lbs.
From college: 265 lbs. Today: 300 lbs.

In high school Jay lettered in
basketball, football and wrestling.

Jay first learned he had
diabetes when he was 12.

Jay has never been hospitalized or missed
a down of football with any diabetes complication.

Jay broke his right hand in the second game
of his senior season, but went on to start
every game that year. (He snapped the ball
lefthanded in one game!)

*  *  *  *  *

Parents no doubt were just as intrigued as their children by the diet of a 300-pound NFL lineman and the blood testing regimen he followed to ensure that his diabetes would not interfere with his play or jeopardize his health during games. Most of them probably never thought twice about the FDA-mandated disclaimers that accompanied this information, or the product references obviously put there by the sponsoring companies.

### JAY'S DIET

|  | Normal Day | Game Day |
|---|---|---|
| Breakfast | 4 scrambled eggs | 6 scrambled eggs |
|  | 1/2 cup grated cheese | 4 pancakes w/syrup |
|  | 4 oz pork sausages | 6-8 oz chicken breast |
|  | 2 slices toast w/jelly | 2 cups fruit/melon |
|  | 2 cups orange juice | 2 cups orange juice |
|  | 2 cups of coffee | 2 cups of coffee |
| Lunch | 4 slices of bread |  |
|  | 10 oz lunch meat | <u>Kick-off</u> |
|  | 1/2 tomato | Gatorade |
|  | 2 lettuce leaves |  |

1 banana

1 orange

2 cups skim milk

1/2 box animal crackers

| Afternoon Snack | Low-fat yogurt | Potato chips |
|---|---|---|
| | 1 cup graham crackers | Water |
| | 2 cups juice | Deli-style sandwich |
| Dinner | 16 oz sirloin steak | 16 oz sirloin steak |
| | Baked potato | Baked potato |
| | w/sour cream | w/sour cream |
| | 3 cups salad | 3 cups salad |
| | w/dressing | w/dressing |
| | 1 large artichoke | 1 large artichoke |
| Evening Snack | 1 pint ice cream | Low-fat yogurt |
| | | Crackers |

Your meal plan should be right for you – right for your diabetes medicine, the kind and amount of exercise you do and any other health concerns you have. See your dietician for more information about diabetes meal planning.

On game day, Jay checks his blood sugar 25 times.

Jay uses his Accu-Chek® Complete™ Monitor to
get information he needs for the control he wants.

Humulin®

human insulin

(rDNA origin)

Each person is different. The amount of insulin you need
depends on your body weight, body build (how much fat
and muscle you have), level of physical activity, daily food
intake, other medicines, emotions, general health and
amount of stress. Consult with your doctor to find the
insulin routine that is best for your needs and lifestyle.

## JAY'S ROUTINE

|  | Normal day | Game day |
|---|---|---|
| 7:00 a.m. |  | Check blood sugar |
| 7:30 | Check blood sugar | Check blood sugar |
|  | Insulin injection | Insulin injection |
| 8:30 |  | Check blood sugar |
| 9:00 |  | Check blood sugar |
| 9:30 |  | Check blood sugar |
| 10:00 |  | Check blood sugar |
| 10:15 |  | Check blood sugar |
| 10:30 | Check blood sugar | Check blood sugar |
| 10:45 |  | Check blood sugar |
| 11:00 |  | Check blood sugar |

| 11:15 | | Check blood sugar |
|---|---|---|
| 11:30 | | Check blood sugar |
| 11:45 | | Check blood sugar |
| 11:50 | | Check blood sugar |
| 11:55 | | Check blood sugar |
| 12:00 p.m. | Check blood sugar | (Kick-off!) |
| | Insulin injection | |
| 1:30-2:00 | | Check blood sugar |
| | | Adjust insulin |
| 3:00 | Check blood sugar | |
| 3:30 | | Check blood sugar |
| 4:00 | | Check blood sugar |
| 5:00 | | Check blood sugar |
| 6:00 | Check blood sugar | Check blood sugar |
| | Insulin injection | |
| 7:00 | | Check blood sugar |
| | | Insulin injection |
| 8:00 | | Check blood sugar |
| 10:00 | | Check blood sugar |
| 10:30 | | Check blood sugar |

Important Safety Information: Potential side effects associated with the use of insulins include low blood sugar, weight gain, low blood potassium, changes in fat tissue at the site of injection, and allergic reactions, both general and local. Starting or changing insulin therapy should be done cautiously and only under medical supervision.

THE GROWTH-CHART poster was distributed to thousands of children across America as part of the Juvenile Diabetes Foundation's Bag of Hope program, by Roche Diagnostics at diabetes camps, at hospitals and schools as part of Jay's speaking appearances, and through doctor's offices. Families who watched Jay and the Colts from Jay's Corner received them, too.

In the spring of 1999, the poster received national acclaim. **"Colts Player's Youth Project Receives Award,"** read the heading on the press release.

"Jay Leeuwenburg, starting center for the Indianapolis Colts, has juvenile, or insulin-dependent, diabetes since age 12. Despite this challenge, he tells children and teens with diabetes that they can achieve their goals as he has done. Now, Leeuwenburg and several collaborators are receiving national recognition for creating a unique method of sharing his positive message across the country.

"The Biomedical Marketing Association recently gave its 1998 Dx Award of Excellence for Patient Marketing and Education to the efforts of Leeuwenburg and the Indianapolis-based companies of Eli Lilly & Company, Roche Diagnostics and The Majestic Group."

The press release, of course, quoted Jay. "We want kids with juvenile diabetes to be like every other kid and fit in. This poster is a great way to make that happen because it creates an opening for kids to educate others about diabetes."

Sue Barlow, marketing manager of education for Roche, was quoted, too. "Kids are highly active, have busy schedules and are often picky eaters. For kids with diabetes, this means sticking to a regular routine of blood-glucose monitoring to maintain good health. The poster helps reinforce that message.

"Jay's positive message and the unusual format made the poster different and cool to kids. We're not surprised by the popularity of the poster."

DESPITE THE accolades, Ingher laments that the poster didn't reach its full potential.

"The more people worked on it and the more they got to know Jay, and the more it came to life, everybody who worked on it knew it was a great project," she said after Jay had been retired for a few years. "Everyone knew it was unique, knew it was dynamic, knew it was great for Roche, and for us.

"But in hindsight, what we didn't do a good job on is this: You look at the yellow rubber bracelet that so many people wore to fight cancer. How could we have make Jay's poster that Lance Armstrong phenomenon? We didn't hit on that.

"After we and Lilly and Roche received the award, it kind of made us realize we probably didn't do enough with it. You know, Jay's a big story. Jay's a positive story. You look at Jay and you would think, 'Gosh darn it, I want to have diabetes, too!

"As big as diabetes is in Jay's life, he could be bigger for diabetes out there in the community. But he is not a self-promoter. He doesn't think what he's done is exceptional. He thinks what he has done is what has been expected. He has never once thought that he achieved more than he should. He does not believe in 'over-achiever." He believes you set a goal for him and he's going to meet it.

"Jay's a story that kind of just eked out in little bits. Maybe continually, but it hasn't had that special, Lance Armstrong effect. Yet his story could have had that effect. That was our disappointment in the poster, the ticket bloc and in the things we did with JDRF."

Other than identifying Jay as the Colts' starting center, the press release made no mention of the football team's involvement in the project. For good reason.

*If you notice, there are no Colts emblems on it. That's because the Colts said they wouldn't help with the poster in any way. I didn't even get any help from the Colts to finance Jay's Corner. We had to buy the season tickets out of our own pocket to make that work.*

*They didn't promote players unless they were exactly who they wanted and exactly how they wanted. They never wanted a player to feel that he had leverage against the team.*

*Their view was, if I became too popular then it would be harder for them to make a business decision to get rid of me. Which obviously I think is the biggest load of bull.*

Whether that thinking was prudent or flawed, it played out as the Colts anticipated in 1999. The award was announced in late April. Four months later, Jay had been released and was off to join his new team, the Bengals, while the Colts defended the decision to unhappy fans.

"Just like Jay's Corner," Ingher frowns, "the poster ended when we left Indianapolis. So did our relationship with Lilly and Roche."

But at least she and Jay know they made a difference. The letters they received leave no doubt.

# CHAPTER 14

# PORTRAIT BY POSTMARK

*"You have become Danny's hero,"*
*wrote one appreciative mother,*
*"and have shown him that this disease*
*doesn't mean your dreams have to end."*

October 4, 1998

Dear Mr. Leeuwenburg,

My son Eric is seven years old and was
diagnosed with juvenile diabetes in September
1996. I don't expect you to remember us, but
Eric and I had the pleasure of meeting you at
the Lilly Tech Center this past summer. You
made a big impression on both of us that night,
but what you did for Eric was more than I
could have hoped for.

Prior to your presentation Eric had asked my
husband and me that we keep his diabetes a
secret when school started this year. I tried to
explain to Eric that this was not possible but
that we would do our best to keep it low-key.
Then a few days before school started, Eric's
new teacher called.

Miss Schreiber wanted to make Eric the Student of the Week to give him the opportunity to tell the kids what information he wanted them to know. This would also help the children understand why Eric would be eating in class. This is where you came in.

When Eric met you he had the pleasure of not only getting your autograph but also having his picture taken with you. Since part of being Student of the Week is bringing in items that you are proud of, he just had to take in the picture of the two of you together.

I was there during Eric's speech just in case any help was needed in answering questions. The talk went wonderfully and the kids were amazed that you had diabetes just like Eric. He told them that you were proof that having diabetes doesn't mean you can't be big and strong. That he can be anything he wants to be!

If you are able to write to the class, I want you to know I would really, really appreciate it. I believe it would make a lifelong impression on the entire class and remind them of the need for compassion and caring in our daily lives.

Respectfully yours,

P.S. Oh, if you just happen to have any autographed pictures lying around, there are twenty-four children in Miss Schreiber's class. Thanks again!

WRITTEN IN every imaginable hand, and sometimes neatly typed, thousands of letters were sent to Jay during his career. They came not only from the cities and states that were home to the NFL teams for which he played, but from all over the country. They came from worried mothers and fathers, anxious grandparents, struggling children and concerned friends.

Some had attended a Colts game in Jay's Corner, or were hoping their name would be drawn soon in the seat lottery. Others had met Jay at Diabetes Camp, or had heard him speak at their school or at a Chicagoland hospital. Still others had only read about him in *Parade Magazine,* on the Internet or in their local newspaper, or had seen him interviewed on public television.

Almost always the letters noted the fateful date when the diagnosis was made. Often they included the person's blood sugar range, the number of tests per day, and the number of injections. Almost without fail there was a request for some kind of token from Jay, an autographed photo or a note of encouragement. Once in a while they asked for more, either a signed football or even a No. 58 jersey.

The pictures sent with many letters matched stories with the earnest faces and sincere smiles of kids next door or down the street, everywhere in America. The stories themselves painted the composite portrait of everyone touched by diabetes, and the fears, challenges and realities they share.

POSTMARK, MILWAUKEE, WI:

Since Danny was 4 years old, he's had a dream of growing up to become a professional football player. On the day he was diagnosed, he said to me, 'I guess there goes my dream of playing professional football when I grow up.' In an emotional phone conversation with a friend of mine, I went on to tell her how crushed my son was. She came to visit him with a Rufus Bear in one hand and your growth chart in the other! That huge poster now hangs on his bedroom wall where he can see it every night before he falls asleep and every morning when he wakes up. You have become his hero and have shown him that this disease doesn't mean your dreams have to end.

POSTMARK, DEPEW, NY:

What words can describe the feeling I still get when I think of my son looking up at you? The relief and understanding that filled his eyes when you spoke with him about feeling the insulin go into your body is something I won't soon forget. I don't know that feeling the way you do - firsthand. Please let us return the favor the next time you're in Buffalo. Our son would love to treat you to a dish of chocolate ice cream!

POSTMARK, FAYETTEVILLE, OH:

It is important to let you know that you have
given me, the parent, hope.  Hope that my son
will be able to experience the fun of sports that
I enjoyed; hope that he can, if he chooses,
accomplish great things, even very great physical
things, in spite of the hurdles in front of him.
You have restored my hope

POSTMARK, SOUTH DAYTONA, FL:

Thank you for pointing our daughter in the
right direction.  She was diagnosed when she
was 3.  We were recently in our doctor's office
in Orlando, and we saw your life-size poster.
My daughter found that to be very interesting.
Well, it wasn't 5 days later when, while channel-
surfing, we stumbled upon the PBS show where
they were interviewing you.  It kept her
attention and she realized that playing sports
can be accomplished with care.  She has been
hospitalized 6 times over the past year.  And
most often it has been after heavy activity.  I
think just hearing it and seeing it come from
you makes her believe that she can do what all
other children do, just with a little extra care.
We are really looking forward to the watch that
will check her system and pass on the warnings
if it sees trouble.  That alone will make her day
(she hates to poke her finger).  We just hope
that the insurance will find this as necessary as

we do; currently they don't pay for Lifescan supplies, so this may fall in the same category. Thank you for the positive outlook on life. I think more shows like that one would be nice. It makes our daughter realize she's not alone.

POSTMARK, INDIANAPOLIS IN:

"I have an 8-year-old son who went to diabetic summer camp this week. While there he received one of your posters, and he was really excited about it. He is currently involved in every sport he can play: baseball, flag football, basketball and soccer. I think my wife and I are more excited about your poster than he was. We have been telling him that he can do anything he wants to as long as he keeps his sugar levels under control. This gives us confidence that we can help him achieve whatever he desires, as long as we teach him the discipline he will need to overcome this obstacle in his life."

POSTMARK, CHICAGO, IL:

(March 6, 1998) It was great seeing you at Lutheran General. As a mother of a 7-year-old who was recently diagnosed a diabetic, your talk was very uplifting to me. To be there in person and hearing your story - gave me more strength. At this stage it is still very new to

us, and my son has had some tough days,
meaning his 'attitude.' And during your talk I
saw him smile at times, so I'm hoping your
speaking to us has helped his attitude. He smiled
when you said you used an accu-check because
that's what he uses.

(March 7, 1998)   Just another short note.
Today my son had his first indoor soccer game.
To my surprise, on his own he prepared some
Gatorade to have on hand, and also remembered
to take his Accu-check. He checked his BS
before, during and after the game. Seeing him
in the gym hall doing that accu-check on his
own assured me that your speech made a
difference in his life. Thanks so much.


POSTMARK, ANCHORAGE, AK:

I am sixteen years old and in April I was
diagnosed with Type I diabetes. I thought all
hope was lost for me to ever do anything
'athletic' in life (I really like to play football and
basketball) until I read an article on the Internet
about you, and it said that you have diabetes.
Somehow that made things easier for me to know
that someone who is diabetic has no problem
playing football (especially on the OL!). Now
don't get me wrong; I don't want anything out of
you. I just wanted to thank you for being such
a good role model for me. That's about it.

POSTMARK, SAN DIEGO, CA:

I am a School Nurse at a large (1100 students)
elementary school here in San Diego. Two of
my male students have diabetes. When I am
discussing their disease with them, they always
say, 'Why do I have diabetes?' and 'Can I play
sports?' If you could send a letter that I can
share with them, I know that you would have a
great impact to help them know that their
disease should not prevent them from attempting
anything in life.


POSTMARK, SCOTTSDALE, AZ:

My eleven-year-old granddaughter was diagnosed
in February 1998, at the age of nine. She has
to test herself 5 or 6 times a day and take four
insulin shots daily Her blood sugar ranges from
a low of 50 to above 400. My daughter is
exhausted just taking care of her, and she has
two other daughters. I am preparing a
'Scrapbook of Hope' of special people, like
yourself, for my granddaughter. Would you be
so kind as to send an autographed picture and a
short note of encouragement?

INGHER SPENT several hours each week, opening, reading and sorting the letters that poured in to the P.O. box she and Jay had set up to handle the volume of mail. Jay tried to read them all, but she would separate the ones she felt he should definitely not miss, highlighting sections that were particularly touching or children who might benefit most from a role model like Jay.

No letter, though, was ever ignored. Everyone who wrote to Jay received a personalized response.

Hello. Let me introduce myself, the letter began.

My name is Jay Leeuwenburg, and I am the starting (position at the time) for the (team at the time). And I, too, am an insulin-dependent diabetic. I was diagnosed with juvenile diabetes when I was 12 years old. I am writing to share with you a little insight on the ups and downs of our disease, and to remind you that you too can follow your dreams and accomplish anything you set your mind to accomplish. Look at me, I am a successful professional athlete, living a very healthy and happy life, on and off the field.

It takes great determination and dedication to become a professional athlete, and it takes even more hard work and discipline to accomplish that as an athlete with juvenile diabetes. You bet, I had ups and downs, and that wasn't just my blood sugar. And just as I have learned to allow my diabetes to become a positive influence in my life, I know that you can, too.

It takes a lot of patience and a lot of trial and error, but if you choose to work with your diabetes rather than against it, you will be able to live a very happy and productive life. My motto: Be in control of your diabetes. Don't let your diabetes control you. You are not alone. Many very successful people live with this disease every day, and so can you.

Enclosed is a picture to remind you that you, too, can do and be whatever you choose. All it takes is hard work and determination. Remember Jay says, "Yes I Can! Yes You Can!"

Your friend,

Jay Leeuwenburg

*When I would go to these health fairs, schools or hospitals, I always tried to have my talk educate the audience. I really tried to impart some of my trials and some of the tribulations and some of the expertise I've learned from my years of living with this disease and being in fortunate circumstances.*

*I would tell each group, 'I've told you all about my life with diabetes, and hopefully you've learned from it. But I can also learn from your life experiences, too. Since I've taken this time to tell you about my life, I would really, really like to know about you. So if you'll write me, I will guarantee to send you something in return.'*

*It was truly a form letter and an autographed 8 by 10 picture. Form letter sounds totally impersonal, but it wasn't. First, I wrote it myself. Second, we addressed it to each kid, personally by name, and I signed every one myself. And if there was such a specific question that you could tell would really help someone out, I'd hand write the answer on top of my letter to them.*

*Someone who is going to take the time to write you a letter, they have a big investment. They're seeking something. If a picture that I could give you, and some words of encouragement, can change your life, I'll still do it to this day.*

*Now, if you're reading the book, and you say, 'Well, he didn't give me a picture,' I did my best. I will guarantee there's somebody I didn't get a picture to. I may have lost some in the thousands of letters I received. But I honestly tried my best.*

*And the other thing I feel really proud of is that I didn't hire somebody to answer the letters for me. Ingher and I personally read and answered every piece of mail I received.*

*Ingher definitely helped me with the addressing and stuffing. At the very beginning, before we got smart, we even paid for all the postage. When it got to be too much, we went to the teams and said, 'This is fan mail. Will you at least postmark it for us?'*

READING EMOTIONAL letter after emotional letter would eventually take its toll on most people. But for the same reason Jay and the JDRF weren't the best fit, he and Ingher were able to resist the natural inclination to respond sympathetically.

"You don't want to sound cold and say these letters don't touch you at the same level," Ingher explains, "but those are the ones that almost need tough love. As Dr. Wolff said, the ones that accept it, the ones that take responsibility – and it has to be both the parents and the child – those are the ones that are going to succeed.

"And you can't do that for them. It's almost like an addiction, or anything in which people have to choose the right path. They have to make those choices. No matter how much you wish it; how much you want it for them; how much you do for them; it's not going to happen until they do it for themselves.

"There are a lot of parents of children with diabetes who are looking for that miracle. Jay's message is not professing a miracle. It is out there communicating how to deal with challenges in your life. It is not giving false hope. It is not saying there is an easy way out. It is saying, 'If you put the effort in, if you're committed, if you're educated, if you takes the necessary steps, you will succeed.'

"There were always going to be kids who were going to be successful at managing their disease. What Jay inspired was for these kids to want more than just managing their disease. He inspired them to join that basketball league, to go out with their friends. He inspired parents to let their kids have the responsibility of having that sleepover that they might not otherwise have let their children have. He inspired children to be children, and parents to be parents of children, not parents of diabetic children.

"Unfortunately, or fortunately – and this is where, Dr. Wolff was so powerful for me – you know what the result will be from day one. It can be predicted by the parents' response to that initial diagnosis.

"If it is the woe is me, the guilt-ridden, how is this possible, what could we have changed – those are the families that struggle through it. If it's the family that says OK, thank God we know what is wrong with you, we can do this, we can work with these guidelines, we can make this work – those are the ones that succeed. It would be interesting to me to know on that day of diagnosis how that family reacted, because I think it's almost black and white.

"The ones who have responded best to Jay are the ones who wanted to hear what he was saying. A lot of people don't want to hear what Jay is saying. They don't want to hear that it's hard work. They don't want to hear that there's not a day off. They don't want to hear that there's no reward for good behavior. They are looking for that miracle that, right now, is not out there."

Tough love notwithstanding, as they shared the time-consuming process of reading all the letters they received, Ingher or Jay often would pause, look at the other, and say, "Oh my goodness. You've got to read this one."

POSTMARK, FREDERICK, MD:

My son Jonathan, who is now 17, was also
diagnosed with diabetes at 12. Unfortunately he
does not have the same attitude you have with
diabetes. He is letting this control his life
instead of him controlling it, as you say. I
don't know if you have the time, but I was
wondering, if possible, if you could drop him a
note telling him that one can live a normal and
even extraordinary life such as yourself with
diabetes. Being a mom and trying to help my
son get out of his slump, I am trying anything
that may help him realize that he can have a
long and great life in spite of this problem. He
has tried to commit suicide three times, as he is
letting this be such a burden for him. He does
not see anything beyond diabetes.

POSTMARK, TERRE HAUTE, IN:

I have a friend with childhood diabetes. She was
diagnosed when she was 11, and is now 28. She
has had a hard time adjusting to this, and has
isolated herself from everyone, even family. I
met her at Indiana State when she was a student
there. She is undergoing eye surgery and may
have lost sight in one eye. She just needs a big
dose of encouragement from someone around her
who understands. You sound like a fighter, and
she needs some fighting spirit right now.

POSTMARK, CINCINNATI, OH:

I have a nephew who is 13 years old.  He just
found out he has diabetes.  He spent a week in
Children's Hospital.  They said he was close to
dying when he was taken in.  He is a very
athletic boy.  He loves to play all sports.  Now
he is afraid he won't be able to play them
anymore.  He is the only boy in his school that
has diabetes.  Some of his (so-called) friends told
him they couldn't be his friend anymore because
he has a disease.


POSTMARK, CROOKSVILLE, OH:

On September 29, 1998 my son was diagnosed
with Juvenile Diabetes at the age of 8.  I will
never forget that day.  It changed my little boy
and our whole family.  We live in rural Perry
County.  The small school he attends has never
had to deal with anything like diabetes.  I
thought we got everyone educated last year and
they understood about diabetes, but I'm finding
out different.  He doesn't like to talk about his
diabetes or feel different from the other kids.
The teacher has made him feel very different
many times.

POSTMARK, INDIANAPOLIS, IN:

My sixth grade year I did a science fair project
on blood sugars and insulin.  I won third place.
I feel my health class didn't stress that many
people could have diabetes and not know it.  In
our book there is at least two pages for every
major disease, but there is only two paragraphs
about diabetes.  I was on our school volleyball
team and my coach wouldn't play me because he
was afraid I would go low.  Only he didn't know
I had a high-energy, high calorie snack before
every game.  I confronted him about this and he
said he just hadn't figured out my strong suit
yet, when everyone on the team knew I was
one of our best servers.  How do you do it?

POSTMARK, KETTERING, OH:

I am 16 years old.  I am a starter on the
varsity field hockey team.  I have played field
hockey for 5 years, and I hope to continue to
play field hockey through college as well.  When
I was three years old, I contracted diabetes
mellitus.  I take 2-3 shots a day and take my
blood glucose level morning, lunch and dinner.
After high school I plan on pursuing a career as
a pediatrician or a career in culinary arts.  I
want to help children who have diabetes better
understand what diabetes is, and how they can
take care of it while they are doing whatever
they want to do.  My mother is a little over-

protective when I stay the night at my friends' houses. She calls at like 1 in the morning to see what my sugar is. I would think that after 13 years of having diabetes, she would've learned to trust me to take care of my diabetes.

POSTMARK, BIG SPRING, TX:

My nephew is ten years old and has had diabetes for four years. He is beginning to play sports, and is feeling more than ever that diabetes makes him different and unable to compete and participate like other children. My nephew knows no children, and very few adults, with diabetes.

POSTMARK, WEYMOUTH, MA:

I found out that I have Type 2 Diabetes two months ago, and at first thought my life was done. Thanks to you and others that share their experiences, I find that I'm going to be fine and enjoy my life with my wife and five-year-old daughter.

NO LETTER Jay received throughout his career summarizes all that he stands for better than one postmarked Lemont, IL. It was one of very few that did not come from a diabetic or a parent or friend of a diabetic.

Dear Jay:

I graduated from Kirkwood in 1989 and was on the wrestling team during your senior year. It was during this time that I learned about your experiences with diabetes and of the courage you displayed while hospitalized.

I was reading the November 21 edition of Parade Magazine, which was featured in the Chicago Tribune, when I noticed your picture in a column that dealt with diabetes. I have been following your career since you were in Chicago and then Indianapolis.

I think that it is super that you try to create a greater awareness of diabetes. As a teacher, coach and an athlete, I think that it is important for kids to know how to control this disease. One of my good mates that I play rugby with also has diabetes. I think that if he would have known of a pro athlete to model himself after, he would have taken better care of himself as a young athlete. It is only now, at the age of 28 that he is really monitoring his sugar levels and watching his diet.

As always, you are proving to be a leader, not only on the field, but off the field as well.

# CHAPTER 15

# CORA AND KATE

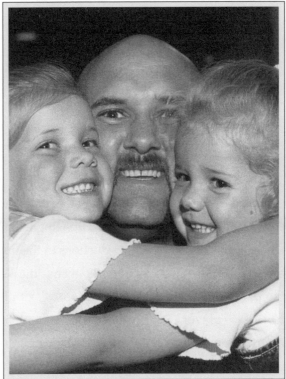

Photo courtesy of Juvenile Diabetes Research Foundation

*Jay's diabetes was never an issue
when he and Ingher decided to start a family.
If Cora or Kate inherits the disease, "they're living
with the best role model," Ingher says.*

PAUL BROWN was an innovator, widely considered the greatest in football history. He conceived the draw play; put face masks on helmets; initiated the practice of studying game films; and was the first coach to call plays from the sidelines, utilizing what he called "messenger guards" to deliver his instructions to the huddle.

When he founded his namesake team, the Cleveland Browns, to play in the new All-America Football Conference in 1946, the first player he signed was a tailback from Northwestern named Otto Graham. And the first thing he did with Graham was convert him into a T-formation quarterback. Graham proceeded to become, many believe, the greatest quarterback of all time.

Elected to the Pro Football Hall of Fame in 1965, Graham led the Browns to championships all four years of the All-America Conference's existence, and to three National Football League titles after the two leagues merged in 1950. His performance in the 1954 NFL Championship Game, when he passed for three touchdowns and ran for three more in a 56-10 victory over the Detroit Lions, remains the greatest single performance in the history of pro football championship games.

Brown himself was dumped by Art Modell in 1963 after Modell won a battle with Brown over ownership of the team. But he founded his second NFL franchise, the Cincinnati Bengals, in 1968, the year after he joined Graham in the Hall of Fame. Those who knew him well always said it was no coincidence that his second franchise had the same initials as his first, nor was it a surprise that his new team's colors were orange and black, the black being as close as he could come to the orange-and-brown contrast of the team he lost.

Unfortunately for Jay, Paul Brown coached the Bengals only through the 1975 season. His final team went 11-3, giving him 222 pro coaching victories to go with 112 defeats and 9 ties. He continued to run the club as general manager until his death, and saw the Bengals play in two Super Bowls. He died at the age of 82 in August 1991, just as defending national champion Colorado was preparing for Jay's senior season.

By the time Jay signed with the Bengals just days before the start of the 1999 NFL season, Paul Brown's standard of excellence was as distant a memory as his steeled glare. Son Mike Brown had been in charge for eight mediocre seasons, during which Cincinnati's best showing was 8-8 and the Bengals' overall record was a dismal 39-89.

*I ended up going to Cincinnati because I thought I was going to have a very good opportunity to start. It was also beneficial because it was all of a 90-minute car ride from Indianapolis. We kept the house in Indianapolis and I commuted every other weekend. Ingher and the girls stayed there.*

*When I reported to the Bengals, I was surprised by what a shambles the organization was in.*

*Literally, they had a box of used jock straps, and if you wore out your jock strap, you went to a cardboard box and your equipment guy told you to pick one out that was your size that somebody else has already worn. They wouldn't even buy you or give you a new jock.*

*It was so bad that KiJana Carter, who had spent his whole career there, had had it – so much so that he bought new towels for all the guys to dry off with because the towels they had wouldn't fit around anybody's waist. They were so cheap, the towels were too small.*

*In the middle of it you had Carl Pickens looking like a total jerk because he wanted to be traded. It was a lot like Corey Dillon, who did the same thing in 2003 and was branded a malcontent. Corey did okay with the Patriots when they won the Super Bowl the next year.*

*With revenue sharing in the NFL, Mike Brown in my opinion just had no incentive to have a good team. It would actually cost him more money if the Bengals got into the playoffs than it would to be 8-8 and have the city still fairly excited.*

*In my experience, the NFL is not the only source of income for many owners. You get a lot of people who have a lot of money who want to prove they can have the best product in whatever field that is.*

*Lamar Hunt was going to be the best in the silver business that he could be. And he was. Because I was drafted by Kansas City, I got to know their feeling. They're going to put the best product they can out there.*

*In Chicago the attitude was, 'We're going to be a reflection of the city. We're hard-nosed, we're tough, we're going to fight and claw and show you that Midwest grit.' Indianapolis was a difficult city because they weren't the Baltimore Colts. There was an identity crisis.*

*And in Cincinnati, it was no longer Paul Brown. It was his son Mike.*

*Mike Brown knew how to make money, but he didn't know how to win football games. Or, more accurately, he didn't particularly care if he won football games.*

*If I had been okay just playing for the money, I probably could have been okay in that city. But after my eighth year, being in Cincinnati and going 4-12 after two straight three-and-thirteens in Indianapolis, it was becoming less and less fun. I wasn't going to play just for the money, so I wanted to get out of there.*

*Money in the NFL means a particular club thinks you are a good player. Who they chose to value at Cincinnati with big contracts was baffling to me. Would I have loved a big contract? Absolutely. But it wasn't going to happen.*

*So if that wasn't going to be the case, and I had told
myself I'm not going to play just for the money, then I
wanted to go to a winner. I wanted to go to a team that I
realistically felt was going to have a chance for that elusive
Super Bowl ring. Because at that point, after my eighth
year, I started understanding that, you turn 30 and
suddenly you're an old man in the NFL.*

*After the season when I was a free agent again, the
responses I was getting through my agent from other teams
told me how I was viewed in the league. My time was starting to run out and I needed to give it one last chance.*


THE OPPOSITE of Mike Brown in the NFL, circa Y2K, was Daniel
Snyder.

Snyder dropped out of college, built a nearly billion-dollar
telephone marketing conglomerate that operated in 12 countries,
then bought the Washington Redskins from the estate of Jack
Kent Cooke – all by the age of 34. One year after outbidding
Cooke's son to acquire the team, Snyder decided to try the
George Steinbrenner approach to building a champion.

The new owner committed more than $115 million to long-
term contracts for big-name free agents. Jay had auditioned for
the morning sports and CU sideline reporter job at KOA radio in
Denver, and had been told a contract was on its way, when the
Redskins asked him if he wanted to come to Washington. They
were on his short list of teams he wanted to play for. He signed
a two-year deal.

In Las Vegas, the Stardust and Hilton Sports Books declared Washington the Super Bowl favorite going into the 2000 season. The most expensive roster in NFL history was the biggest story in the league – every step (and misstep) reported in the context of Snyder's extravagance and whether or not it would succeed.

"Redskins fans are so disenchanted with Washington's $100 million underachievers that they booed owner Daniel Snyder during halftime ceremonies Monday night," wrote one NFL columnist. "A 3-0 start against the softer part of the schedule was expected; indeed the first three opponents have gone 1-5 against teams other than the Redskins. But Washington is 1-2 and reeling."

Five straight victories followed, and it began to look as though Snyder yet might realize the return he was seeking on his investment. But a 9-7 loss to New York on December 3 – the fourth in five games following the winning streak – dropped Washington's record to 7-6.

The Associated Press began its report of that game with, "The New York Giants finally won as underdogs, returning to first place in the NFC East with a defense that turned the big-money Washington Redskins from favorites to flops." Four paragraphs later, "The Redskins (7-6) are on the verge of elimination, and coach Norv Turner is on the brink of losing his job."

*We had purchased, under Daniel Snyder, what we all thought was a Super Bowl team. It was in everyone's mind who signed a free agent contract that year. It was reminis-*

*cent of what we all grew up with –when the 49ers bought a Super Bowl.*

*The Redskins had signed Bruce Smith. They had signed Deion (Sanders). They had Stephen Davis as the running back. Brad Johnson was the quarterback. We had Michael Westbrook, James Thrash, Stephen Alexander. We had Marco Coleman, and still had Darrell Green.*

*We had, in our opinion, the best talent. I really felt confident that was going to be the year we were going to go places.*

*There are a lot of reasons it didn't happen. We were the team to beat, and it's a long season. If you're going to get every team's best shot, it wears you down.*

*Brad Johnson did not have a very good year. Stephen Davis did not have a very good year. Brad later won a Super Bowl with Tampa Bay as their quarterback. And Stephen Davis, with Carolina, made it to the Super Bowl. So these are guys who could produce. It really hurt to have two of your main offensive guns not have good years.*

*And at times there definitely were chemistry issues. It was not talked about, but there were rumblings about who was making the decisions. Was it Norv Turner or was it Daniel Snyder? We as players expected to win; we got everyone's best shot. And then there was the uncertainty about 'Who am I playing for?' There was no clear line.*

*Having said all that we were still in the playoff hunt when they fired Norv Turner and replaced him with Terry Robiskie. That was a huge mistake.*

*Terry's style was to come in and change too many things. He wanted to make too many offensive changes in a short amount of time. We didn't have time to practice and master them.*

*And his motivation approach was to yell and scream, which was different than Norv. There were too many differences in style, both personality and playbook-wise, with only three games left in the season. We lost the next two before we won a game under Terry. So we finished 8-8.*

*To this day, with the amount of veteran leadership and playoff experience we had on that team, if we had gone 9-7 and made it to the playoffs, I believe that team was built to win in the playoffs. It didn't matter how we got in; had we gotten into the playoffs, we could have gone a long way. I think to a certain extent every one of our guys may have been saving up a little to make that playoff run; and they saved too much.*

*It was another very difficult season for me. When Norv got fired and Terry Robiskie came in to coach the last three games, it was miserable. Those were the hardest three games of my career. The first one, at Dallas, was the worst.*

*Dallas and the Redskins, based on my experience, seems to be a bigger rivalry than Green Bay and Chicago. They truly hated each other. We went to Dallas, and long story short, I got kicked out of the game.*

*We dressed six linemen, and I went against Alonzo Spellman, who was a first round draft pick out of Ohio State for the Bears the same year I was drafted. I didn't like him in Chicago and let him know it. I thought he was a prima donna, overrated, very immature and making way too much money for what he did. I didn't respect Alonzo. I didn't like anything about him, and he knew I didn't like him.*

*So I'm playing for the Redskins and he's playing for the Cowboys. On the very first play of the game, Dallas ran a line stunt and their defensive end, Ebeneezer Ekuban, came down and intentionally, to my mind, tried to blow my knee out. Alonzo held me up, while Ekuban just put his helmet right in my knee.*

*It's one of the only times I can remember someone truly got into my head. I prided myself on being a smart player. But the rest of the game I was truly trying to hurt the guy who tried to blow out my knee.*

*Eventually, I knocked him out. He stumbled off the field and didn't show up for about three series. They ran the same line stunt and, I saw him coming and just lit him up. So there was a lot of jawing and extracurricular activity in the game.*

*A little later, Alonzo was rushing the passer and I went to cut him. He took exception to it. One of his physical attributes that made him a first-rounder is he has some of the longest arms I ever played against. He got up and grabbed my face mask with one hand, and there are two officials right next to me. So I put my arms down and started screaming and yelling and cursing at him, and he started punching me. Never did I retaliate.*

*They threw us both out of the game. I couldn't believe I was thrown out of the game. It was the only game I was* *ever thrown out of, and to this day, I didn't do anything wrong. I was fined $12,500 by the league, but that was later rescinded, so the league agreed in hindsight that I didn't do anything wrong or illegal that would merit my getting thrown out of the game.*

*I do not know, and never met, Jerry Jones, the owner of the Cowboys. But he was on their sideline that day, and I vividly remember, as I'm being escorted off the field by armed policemen, looking at the Jumbotron and seeing Jerry Jones hugging Alonzo Spellman and telling him what a great job he did.*

*We're in Dallas and they loved it that this folk hero, Alonzo Spellman, did this. I called Ingher from the locker room, and, literally, I've got two guys with guns watching me get undressed to make sure I don't go back on the field. I remember screaming at them, 'I'm not going back! Give me some privacy'*

*The next day Robiskie blamed our loss specifically on me for getting kicked out of the game. We lost 32-13, and he's blaming the loss on me – with my not having done anything to get thrown out of the game! At that point I was ready to retire from the game. I had had enough.*

CORA ISABELLA Leeuwenburg was born during Jay's fifth year in the league, soon after he signed with the Colts. Her sister Kate Louise came along two years later in the spring of '98, the same year the "Yes I Can" poster was born.

The possibility that their children might inherit diabetes from their father is something Ingher and Jay discussed, but it never caused them to hesitate when they decided to get serious about having a family.

"Statistically, they have a 33% chance of having it," Ingher says. "But it wasn't something that had an impact on us to say we weren't willing to risk having a baby. As I said to Jay, if it does happen, they're living with the best role model."

Jay's locker was an easy one to find. Just look for the pictures of his family. The closest he came to living a season away from Ingher and the girls was that year in Cincinnati, when he commuted to Indianapolis every other weekend. The next year, they rented a house in the nation's capital.

One of his favorite memories – and possibly the only really good one from his season in Cincinnati – is seeing his girls cuddle with the Bengal tiger mascot at the 50-yard line in Cinergy Field before a game. What he enjoyed most about Washington was seeing his girls react to the White House, the landmarks and the museums.

Family has always been a priority for Jay. It is the importance of his family that shaped Jay's future after his Redskins experience.

*I was brought in, according to the Redskins, not to be a starter. So my base salary reflected that. I said that was fine, but if they do that, then I would like incentives in my contract, not only monetarily but also for playing time.*

*If I played more than 50 percent of the downs, I voided the second year of my contract and I became an unrestricted free agent – thinking if we make the playoffs and I'm a starter, they're going to want me back, and I'll be able to get a better contract.*

*I ended up playing 85% of the downs, but we went 8-8, didn't make the playoffs and they fired the coach. So that strategy didn't work.*

*Having gone to CU, whenever I was a free agent I always had my agent call the Broncos and say, 'What do you think of Jay Leeuwenburg?' I respected Alex Gibbs, the Broncos' offensive line coach, because he was always honest about his feelings. He said, "I do not like him as a player. He will never play for the Denver Broncos as long as I'm here." I didn't fit his mold of player.*

*Alex had retired, and Rick Dennison was the offensive line coach. Rick Dennison loved me as a player. He thought I'd fit perfectly in the system. So I signed a free agent contract with the Broncos.*

*But then Alex Gibbs comes out of retirement and I'm under contract. So I went to Mike Shanahan and said, Mike, if you're just going to cut me, don't make me go through another training camp. If you have no interest in keeping me, then I'll just be done.*

*I go through training camp, the whole thing. And Rick Dennison tells me if it was up to him I would have made the team, but Alex Gibbs cut me. He was supposed to be part-time, but he was still running the show.*

*I'd had very little contact with Gibbs. He was there maybe half the time. In my opinion I could have been the best lineman they had, and he still wasn't going to think I was any good. The day Gibbs came back, they signed David Diaz-Infante, a Gibbs guy, and he made the team. I naively thought I could still make the team. I thought I could change his mind.*

*So I go into Mike's office, literally with the pink slip, and he tells me what a good camp I had, and tells me, here are four teams that have contacted him that have a roster spot for me. He tells me that they've looked at me all pre-season.*

*He says these teams are really interested in me – I can go here, here, here or here. I think it was Detroit, the Raiders, the Chargers and Arizona. At which point I looked at him and told him, "I already told you that if you were going to do this, this is the only team I want to play for."*

*The girls were getting to the age when they would be in school. My oldest, Cora, was already accepted to Colorado Academy; she was attending school. And that makes a difference. Education is extremely important for our children. We're not going to use our kids as little toy things and run all over the country.*

*We knew that at whatever point it happened, we wanted to retire in Colorado. Ingher is from Colorado, and I went to school here. We wanted to be around the mountains; we love the area. So I basically told him to go fly a kite.*

*I told him, 'If it makes you feel better to tell me you prepped me so I could audition for other teams, that's fine.*

*But that's not why I was here. I was here to make this team and to play for this team.'*

*I told him that I really did not respect him and did not think it was fair the way he handled it. And that was the end of the meeting.*

*If someone had gotten hurt, or had Alex Gibbs stayed retired, I would have been a Denver Bronco. But you look at it from Mike Shanahan's point of view. He has no history with me. I don't know the relationship he had with Alex Gibbs, but it obviously was tumultuous. But they still valued him as a member of their coaching staff.*

*So it makes sense. Did I like it? Absolutely not. Did I feel like I was lied to? Yes. But it's Shanahan's right as a head coach. It makes sense for him to back his coach and not me, an unknown entity.*

*The day I was cut from the Broncos, we were in a house in Highlands Ranch, renting. I remember Ingher saying, in a very positive way, "If you still feel this need to be able to play, then go out to L.A. and play. We'll support you, but the girls and I are going to stay." They'd moved three times in three years.*

*I couldn't see myself being that selfish. I had made a commitment to my family that I wasn't going to move. I was not going to another city and have my family in Denver. I always had my family with me.*

FOUR YEARS after he walked out of Mike Shanahan's office, and in the process walked out of the NFL for good, Jay still had never heard of GAMESOVER.org. Which is positive. He was unfamiliar with it because, unlike the hundreds of ex-NFL players it is designed to help, Jay was able to move into everyday life without crisis.

In his Welcome Letter, founder Ken Ruettgers introduces GAMESOVER.org – "Where a New Season Begins" as "the first and only non-profit web site dedicated to serving and meeting the transitional needs of (NFL) players when they leave the game."

A key member of the offensive line that opened holes for Marcus Allen and bought time for quarterback Rodney Peete while they were collegiate stars at the University of Southern California, Ruettgers was drafted in the first round by Green Bay in 1985, and became a celebrity in that football-crazy town.

He played 12 seasons for the Packers; tasted Super Bowl victory; and was the offensive unit's most valuable player in 1989. Injuries forced him to retire during the 1996 season.

Ruettgers was different than many NFL players when they reach the end of their careers, in that he had completed his degree and had begun a second career in the off-seasons. Yet he was just like them, too, in that he could not adjust to life away from the regimen, discipline, camaraderie, competition, fame and fortune of pro football.

In a segment of HBO's Sports with Bryant Gumbel in January 2005, Ruettgers said the toughest thing for him early in retirement was "getting up in the morning to take a shower." He said he would think to himself, "What do I have to live for? My best days are gone." He told of meeting a Green Bay fan on the street and hearing the fan say, "Wait a minute. Didn't you used to be Ken Ruettgers?" He told Gumbel he answered, "I think I still am."

Ruettgers looked for support, but found none. He wondered if he was an exception, and found he was far from alone in his distress. "There was an epidemic out there," he told Gumbel.

When he looked more closely, Ruettgers learned that the lives of ex-NFL players were filled, to an alarmingly greater degree than the general population in America, with business failure, personal bankruptcy, divorce, domestic violence, substance abuse, physical disability, anger, isolation, depression and suicide. He found purpose in serving others like himself.

While Jay wonders how it could get so bad for so many ex-players, he does understand the adjustment they all face. He experienced it, too.

*I was not very motivated my first year out of pro football. The only thing I really did that was constructive was that I was able to lose some weight. I had made it a priority, for my health and my diabetes, to lose some weight.*

*You have to remember that almost everyone who leaves the game is not wanted any longer. Nobody likes to get fired from their job. I'm as close as you can come to an exception, because it was my decision. But I made that decision because somebody didn't want me.*

*If I had been okay just playing for money in a backup*

role and keeping my mouth shut, I could have stayed in the league for several more years. But that's not why I played. I played football because I loved playing. I didn't play football for the money. I played it because I loved the competition. I loved the game. It absolutely tore me up inside and made it miserable if I wasn't able to play. So a backup role was unthinkable for me.

Leaving pro football was a very different challenge in my life, and the transition was not exactly the smoothest. Mentally it was very difficult to leave. I didn't watch football for a year. I got really angry. I was very conflicted.

I was still arrogant enough to say, 'I should still be playing.' Most people when they're cut and forced to retire, say that. 'Well if I really wanted to, I could be on the team.' But it doesn't matter if you could still play or not, because you're not.

At times I'd be lying if I said you don't miss the paycheck.

The reality is, I once made a commercial with Jim Harbaugh and made more in a weekend than teachers make their first year teaching. You live in a fantasy world. You lose all sense of the value of money.

There are guys in the NFL who, if you're not getting a minimum brand new car a year, it's like, 'What's wrong with you?' You might be getting two or three a year, plus the one you get for doing a TV commercial that's given to you with a free lease for a year. You don't think that lifestyle is ever going to end.

*I was different in that I didn't have two houses, didn't have two mortgages. I didn't get a new car every year. I didn't own $300,000 worth of jewelry. I didn't have an entourage. I didn't have three cell phones and two beepers.*

*Still it's a humongous change in lifestyle when you leave the NFL. We're talking about putting on the brakes, financially. For the first time, you have to be on a budget. You start learning about things you never thought about before.*

*Another thing that really became evident for me was this feeling that, 'I'm not qualified. I have no training for any other vocation except to be hard-nosed and, essentially, beat somebody up.'*

*I think there were several factors that helped me beat the statistics. My dad was the perfect example of life after football; he put it all in perspective. And from age 12, I have had to have the discipline to deal with diabetes. There was something bigger than football in my life. And family is truly important to me.*

*Most of all, I had a great support system. In a loving way, Ingher told me, 'You need to figure out what you want to do. You're 32-33 years old; you've got a lot of living to do. What kind of role and what kind of example are you going to be giving your children if you stay home and do nothing? You're not going to be a productive citizen. You're not going to be someone you value or you want Cora and Kate to value.'*

*So I started thinking about what brought me joy, besides football. With that I started volunteering at my daughters' school.*

# CHAPTER 16

# THIRD GRADE

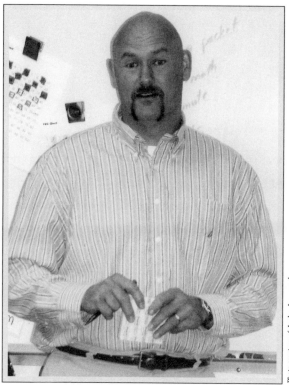

Photo courtesy of Ingher Leeuwenburg

*"Obviously, I never deny I was an NFL player.*
*But I feel I have so much more to offer*
*these students. I want to show them that I am*
*a teacher, somebody they can learn from."*

THE CAMPUS of Colorado Academy occupies 95 acres neighboring Pinehurst Country Club on the southwest edge of Denver. Driving onto the tree-laden grounds is like entering a centuries-old estate in the English countryside, or the campus of a small private college in the East. A visitor quickly senses that this is a place with history, pride and tradition.

C.A., as it's known to those who are familiar enough to speak of it informally, was founded in 1906. That same year, a historic earthquake flattened San Francisco; the volcano Vesuvius devastated Naples, Italy; SOS was adopted as the international distress signal; and Theodore Roosevelt became the first sitting American President to venture outside the United States on an official visit when he went to check on construction of the Panama Canal.

About 200 yards down the lane from the main entrance, the way forks and a sign offers directional choices: right to the Library, Theatre, Athletic Center, Middle School, Upper School and Headmaster's Office; left to the Visual Arts Center and Gallery, Pre-School and Lower School. The Lower School is for students in kindergarten through fifth grade.

C.A. describes itself as "an independent, nonsectarian, coeducational, college preparatory day school that provides exceptional learning opportunities for students from Pre-Kindergarten through twelfth grade." And, referring to its educational program, states: "The integrated, innovative curriculum emphasizes group and individual study of the liberal arts, in addition to experiential learning and community service."

Total enrollment approaches 900. The student-teacher ratio is a tidy 9-to-1, and the average class is 17 pupils. Quality personalized instruction comes, of course, with a hefty price. In 2005, the tab was $9,500 per year for full-day Pre-Kindergarten, $13,450 for Kindergarten, $14,635 for grades 1-5, and $15,425 for grades 6-12.

A year of classes at some colleges and universities is less expensive, but then, you get what you pay for. One hundred percent of C.A.'s students attend four-year colleges, according to C.A. Fast Facts.

Thumbnail profiles of C.A.'s 100-plus teachers are filled with references to master's degrees, post-graduate studies and work at renowned universities around the world. Clearly, this is an accomplished staff. In fact, one of the third grade teachers even played nine years in the National Football League.

When I was being recruited by CU and the other schools, I was going to be an engineer. I was going to build bridges and things like that. But after my second year in school, I met third semester physics, which killed me. I loved the math, but I really had a hard time with the physics of it.

I took a midterm physics exam, and got 19%. But it was graded on a curve, so I got a C. For some reason, the collapse of that hotel balcony in Kansas City in 1981 had stuck with me. Maybe it was because it happened the year I was diagnosed. In any event, I thought of it right away, eight years later, as if it had just happened, when I got my grade on that test.

I thought, 'Well, no wonder! If you can get a 19% and you get a passing grade in physics, I can now see how that happened. I'm not going to go out there and build walkways and bridges, and kill people.'

So I said, 'I'm done.' At that point, I took this logical step: I had taken one English class, and it was fun. I decided I'd be an English major. I graduated in four years, and I got my 3.0 average.

As I've said, in my fifth year, the NCAA had not caught up with athletes who graduate in four years and have a red-shirt year left. I was told by NCAA that I had one option: get into a Graduate School program or be ineligible. So in that fifth year, I was admitted to the Graduate School of Business. But I enrolled in some education classes.

In the back of my mind, it was a profession I thought I might be interested in. I was still truly focused on making *a run in the NFL. But at the same time the reality was, I had to take some classes. So I took some education classes in grad school.*

*The realistic decision that, 'I'm going to make a run at being a teacher' came after I didn't make it with the Broncos. Cora was a kindergartner at Colorado Academy. Part of my retiring was my commitment that I was going to spend more time with my children and my wife.*

CHRIS BABBS and Dick Leeuwenburg had been best friends for more than 40 years by the time Jay's football career came to an end in Mike Shanahan's office on September 2, 2001, just nine days before the 9/11 attacks that shook America to its core values. They still talked regularly, and, with their wives, visited once or twice a year.

Classmates at Stanford, they met as teammates on the freshman football team in 1960. Chris was a tailback who would give up football after one season to concentrate on basketball and track, Dick that offensive lineman who would get a chance to play professionally.

In the years that followed, Dick and Chris roomed together; Chris was Dick's Best Man when he married Jann; Dick and Jann named their first son Chris; Jann and Nancy Babbs, Chris's wife, became close friends, too; and Dick and Jann asked Chris to be Jay's godfather.

While Dick succeeded in business, Chris became an educator of accomplishment. He was named Head of School at

Colorado Academy in 1991, Jay's final season at the University of Colorado, and became Jay's boss a pro career later.

It would be easy to jump to the conclusion that Jay became a member of the C.A. faculty just because Chris was in charge. But that would be incorrect. It's true that the opportunity to explore teaching as a career was there because of it. Jay, though, had to earn the job.

"People could say, oh, gosh, you knew Jay's dad and you sponsored him, and that's why he got a job here," Babbs concedes. "On the contrary, sometimes when you have that influence, it can work against you. Jay underwent higher scrutiny because of it."

*At times I think it has been more difficult in that I've been looked at and scrutinized a little more. Because there can be no sense of preferential treatment.*

*Chris Babbs changed my diapers when I was a baby. I mean, he knew me before I have any memory.*

*I don't think Chris would have advertised that we have that relationship, but I'm sure something was mentioned, like, 'Why don't you give him a shot and see what happens?' I don't know if that door would have been opened had that relationship not been there.*

*I think it was really tough on Chris and my father. What happens if I couldn't make the grade? What happens if I'm not a very good teacher? I get this chance, and then I fail?*

*That could be a huge strain on my father and his best friend for 35 years. There are plenty of parents who don't have the best of children, you know. You want to help your friend, but you don't want to ruin your relationship because you're trying to help his son out. I think he felt a lot of pressure.*

ACTUALLY, BABBS says, it was never an issue. "This just became another phase of our friendship. Dick does not probe into how Jay's doing; he respects the fact that I'm his boss. I'll volunteer some reassuring things once in a while, but he really doesn't ask.

"As every boss does, I've had some boss conversations with Jay. But he doesn't run home and call his dad. Jay respects the friendship and values it, and doesn't ever want it to be a problem."

It all began when Jay signed with the Broncos after Daniel Snyder's hundred-million-dollar Redskins crashed and burned.

"It's very serendipitous," Chris recalls. "Jay and Ingher called me because he was moving back to Denver, and they were looking into the school situation for their girls.

"At first they didn't look into my school. They were just looking for general information about schools and school districts. They didn't even know we were a Pre-K through 12 school; they thought we were a high school.

"Jay didn't come, but Ingher came, visiting from Indianapolis. She came to see me and Nancy, and we brought her over to the C.A. campus. She looked around and said, 'Why not this school?' This is the school Ingher wanted for the girls."

Chris thought no more of it as Jay went through Denver's entire training camp that summer of 2001, only to be one of the Broncos' last cuts. Shortly after Jay's career-ending meeting with Shanahan, the Leeuwenburgs and the Babbs had dinner.

"He was looking for something to do," Babbs recalls. "So I said, 'Why don't you offer to volunteer in a Lower School classroom, in the art classroom?' He met Carole Buschmann that way.

"It was a little test on my own part, I have to admit," Babbs confides. "I wanted to get the feedback from some of our teachers down there. What was he like?

"I had my instincts about teachers. Jay's got the temperament for it. He majored in English in college, so I thought he'd be a great high school teacher – teach high school English and coach. And then I saw him with his girls; he's a wonderful dad, really a natural with that age group. He also has artistic interests – he's been a ceramicist."

Carole Buschmann is from Jay's mom's generation. And she's a lot like Jann: upbeat, breezy personality; artistically blessed and possessing a nurturing acceptance of right-brain independence that enabled her to enjoy Jay much as Jann did and does. Jann was a teacher once, too, though briefly, compared to Carole's almost 25 years.

"Mr. Babbs asked if any of us were going to be working in clay," Carole recalls. 'I said, 'I'll be doing that soon.' So Jay showed up. He was this huge, giant guy, but it was obvious he was a gentle soul.

"I remember I took him to the kiln room, and on the way we passed a group of students. They ignored me, but they saw

him, and four boys were around him in no time. They could tell
by his build he was a football player. I'm such a non entity, and
he stood out.

"I thought, 'This is too cool.' You're always looking for
people who will get kids excited about the arts. It was clear that
he would.

"It was great. He had good ideas about the students. It
was clear he was interested in teaching."

*I wanted to volunteer. I wanted to get back in touch
with my art. So I called the Lower School art teacher,
Carole Buschmann, introduced myself, and asked if I could
volunteer in any way to help her in the Art Department.*

*I had also taken some art classes in college and had
seriously considered opening my own ceramics studio
instead of becoming a teacher. I have a passion for that. I
love it.*

*Carole was extremely gracious, and said, basically, 'I
have no idea who you are. I guess I understand you're
going to have a kindergartner in school here. Let me do
some checking around.' It came about that she said later,
'Why don't you come in on Fridays and we'll get to know
each other, and I'll see what you can do.'*

*I got to see a master teacher. She is just fabulous the
way she is able to manage a classroom and teach art, and
also connect with and light the passion in children.*

*I went in every Friday, and I loved it. I absolutely*

*loved being with the children. It was such a change from*
*the NFL, so different from all the macho, 'this is more*
*important than life itself' mentality that is always spewed*
*at you in all the locker rooms of the NFL.*

*You have the grotesqueness – just the vulgarity – that*
*goes on, the barbarianism of the attitudes, and how it's*
*admired. And then to go into a situation where you have six-*
*year-olds slopping paint on a piece of paper, and it's the best*
*thing ever. There's laughter, and, 'Hey look at my lady bug!'*

*It's what my soul needed. I absolutely loved it. At*
*that point, the seed was planted: 'This is pretty neat. I*
*could see myself doing this.'*

THE SAME year Colorado Academy opened its doors, the United
States Congress established America's eighth national park in
the arid Four Corners region of Colorado, near the point where
the borders of Utah, New Mexico and Arizona come together
with Colorado. It was called Mesa Verde. A connection between
the school and the park developed decades later, and continued
as both approached their 100th anniversaries.

Mesa Verde – "green table" in Spanish – is the land of the
Anasazi, early Native Americans who made their home above
the canyons near what is now the city of Cortez, Colorado, from
roughly 600 to 1300 A.D. During the last century that they
inhabited the area, almost 200 years before Christopher
Columbus discovered the New World, they moved from the top
of the mesas to the canyon walls, perhaps for greater security.

They abandoned the area sometime during the fourteenth century because, archaeologists speculate, drought made it impossible to grow enough food on the mesas to feed the settlement. They left behind a virtual outdoor museum for a way of life that no one after them knew existed for the next five hundred years.

The most noted Western wilderness photographer of the nineteenth century, William Henry Jackson, is the first white man known to have entered a Mesa Verde cliff dwelling. That was in 1874. He named his discovery Two-Story Cliff House. Many other sites were found in the years to follow, including some of today's tourist favorites.

In all, archaeologists have uncovered more than 4,000 sites, including more than 600 cliff dwellings, within Mesa Verde National Park's 52,000 acres. Each year almost a half-million visitors examine these ruins and marvel at the ingenuity, resourcefulness and determination of a people that seems to have vanished before Columbus even knew their continent existed.

The National Park Service also offers numerous educational programs within the park. They attract many school children each year, including some from Colorado Academy.

*There's a program at Colorado Academy in which the fifth grade students go for a week for an extended field study down to Mesa Verde. It's called the Crow Canyon Archaeological Center. It has cabins and a dining center and other things.*

*Two parent chaperones always go along with the*

*classes. You can't have a student in fifth grade and be a chaperone. Since my student was in kindergarten, and they saw the way I acted around students and young children, they asked me if I wanted to do it. I wasn't doing anything else, so I said, 'Sure.'*

*I went, and then I fell in love with these fifth graders for a week. I was responsible for 13 fifth grade boys in my cabin.*

*At this point I started thinking about becoming a teacher a lot more seriously. How could I make a difference in people's lives? Very few men are in elementary education.*

*I spent a week down there, and as soon as we got back, I applied to be a substitute teacher. Because it's a private school, I didn't need to be licensed or certified. I just had to go through the proper background checks.*

*Mrs. Buschmann was great. She actually started letting me take small groups of kids and work with them and actually teach them. Then after the three fifth grade teachers saw that I was really more than a chaperone – that I was almost another teacher – I became a substitute teacher. I subbed three days a week.*

*Almost right away, I said, "How can I go about becoming a teacher?"*

IF TIMING IS everything, as they say, Jay's at C.A. proved to be perfect, both for a new way to become a teacher that was developing at the school, and for openings that were developing but not yet apparent.

"At that same time," Chris Babbs explains, "we were developing an intern program at the school, attached to the alternative certification program of the Colorado Department of Education. One thing led to another, and I thought Jay should apply to that. He did, and we had him as an intern, one of our first interns in the intern program."

The Alternative Teacher Licensure Program was introduced in Colorado in January 1991, shortly after the CU Buffs won their National Championship in the Orange Bowl. The purpose was to address a shortage of qualified teachers at all levels, and it succeeded. Between 450 and 500 "Alternative Teachers" worked in Colorado schools the year of Jay's internship and the year that followed.

"It's a rigorous program," Babbs continues. "You have to have so many practicum hours in classrooms, and you have to cover some additional requirements. You have to have competency areas, and you have to develop a portfolio that you have to present at the end of the year to a school committee with some outside representatives from the state board of education. Jay passed all of those tests with flying colors.

"I thought we were just getting him in a situation to be certified, so he could teach *somewhere*. Talk about going from dinner to an intern program that we just happened to be putting together. Sure enough, the next step, which we never predicted, was that there would be an opening here at C.A."

*I spent the majority of the first semester of my intern-
ship in fifth grade, but I went to first grade for a few days.
I wanted to go down to first grade before I moved there for
second semester so there wasn't this huge man suddenly
teaching those students. I wanted to familiarize them with
who I was.*

*It really helped having my daughter there because
they had seen me as a parent in the community. It also
helped that I had worked with Carol Buschmann because
she teaches all grades. So I was already on the fringes of this
community. There are a lot of parent volunteers anyway at
this school.*

*In fifth grade the attitude is pretty much, 'You're
mature enough to accept when I tell you that you need to do
something. I don't need to repeat myself.' That's part of the
maturing process.*

*I went down to first grade, and it was totally differ-
ent. In ten minutes, I was down there, and I just looked at
this young boy and said something like, 'Didn't I tell you
that you needed to go get a piece of paper or get your note-
book?' It was something like that.*

*He just looked at me and burst into tears. I was just
instantly thinking, 'Oh my gosh, what did I get into?' It
was very humbling.*

*The fifth graders had gotten used to me, and they are
so much more mature. All of a sudden I'm doing first
grade, and I'm thinking, 'Oh my gosh, what am I doing?
I'm going to ruin this child.'*

*At the end of that year a third grade and a fourth grade teaching position became open. So I applied for both.*

*I think it's fairly typical of my personality and my life, that whether it be the NFL or whether it be college, it often-times seems like I'm the luckiest person you've ever seen. It doesn't even look like I have a plan.*

*But I knew somewhere in the back of my mind – there was a reason I took education classes in college; there was a reason I sought out children for my community service.*

JAY WASN'T an automatic choice, even though he obviously enjoyed the advantage of familiarity – his with the school and its faculty, and theirs with him. His godfather's priority steadfastly remained finding the best person for the job.

"We interviewed several candidates for the job," Babbs quickly points out. "Jay had to go down there and interview with the third grade team. I wanted an affirmation from four or five teachers who worked with him, plus the principal, Fran Trujillo. I wanted to know, 'Is he the guy, Fran? Is he the one we would be hiring without these associations?'

"They knew they had my permission to say back to me, 'This is not going to work.' They knew if they did say it was not going to work, I would not push it, because that would have put Jay in an absolutely impossible situation."

By then, though, the volunteer-turned-intern-teacher had grown on everyone who had worked with him.

"There were teachers who saw gifts in Jay that they didn't

have, and they were very complimentary about him: a very natural teacher; good classroom management skills; great sensitivity to the needs of that age group; a very creative and inventive teacher; creates interesting lessons that revert into actual skills the students need to learn but makes those skills more interesting; a good math teacher who had, really, a gift for making mathematics instruction at that level very comprehensible and challenging.

"Carole said he was really quite good. He had a natural touch with the kids. He had a natural teacher's instinct, which is really the excitement you get when you're trying to present something new. And he loved the age group down there."

Carole Buschmann saw something else that really appealed to her, too. She liked it that Jay had competed in the NFL, though not because she loves football or thinks athletes are more than human beings with a special talent.

"As opposed to someone just out of college, Jay had seen people succeed and fail," she explains. "He was part of a mature profession. He understood, and saw first hand, that even though you want something and work hard for it, you might not get it. Whether that's losing a big game, or not making the team, that's a great perspective to be able to pass on to children."

When the hiring decision finally was made, it was the other members of the third grade team who convinced Chris Babbs that he was not leading with friendship's heart.

"The clincher for me," he says, "was that the other two third grade teachers said, 'He will bring great strengths to this team that we don't have now.' One of them who was to be his mentor, a very skilled, experienced teacher, felt she could be helpful to Jay but also felt that there would be some reciprocity. She felt she would learn from him, too."

"So, a happy conclusion. You always like to bring young people to the teaching profession. To have that happen with your best friend's son is great."

*In the beginning, the hardest part for me was that, in the NFL, literally every six-inch step you take, every hand placement you have, is scrutinized. Everything you do, almost to every breath you take, is critiqued. That's what I was used to.*

*After the first week of school, I was ready to have a film review. Tell me what I did well. Tell what I need to improve on. Coach me.*

*But the attitude was more like, 'We hired you because we trust you. We know what you can do. It's okay if you weren't perfect in that one sentence when you were speaking to your students. They got the idea.'*

*It is refreshing that every step and every pen stroke isn't filmed and analyzed. I had 15 years where everything was dissected and analyzed and criticized. Life doesn't have to be that fast. Life doesn't have to be that exaggerated. I'm really enjoying that difference.*

*The adage in the NFL was, if the coach isn't talking to you, that's an indication you are probably out the door. In education, and I believe in most other jobs or professions, they'll speak to you when they feel you need some guidance or assistance. If they don't say anything, you assume things are going well. That took some adjusting.*

*The thing I've come to realize is that having all those little tools and tricks definitely helps to make you a good teacher. But the thing you can't prepare for, and can't coach in a teacher, and that I need to continue to maintain, is my own enthusiasm for teaching and working with the children.*

*It's infectious. When I am excited to be at school and when I am so excited about teaching this subject, that's what the students remember. When I am energetic and I'm ready to go, and I greet the day and I'm excited to see all the students, and I ask them how they're doing, how was their weekend, and what did they do over the summer, and how is their brother – that's what they remember.*

*Yes, they're going to learn how to multiply and how to write cursive. But it can't be overemphasized: if they see me loving to teach, and excited about their advances and when they get a concept or skill, they can feel that energy and enthusiasm. That's one of my strengths: making every student feel special.*

*You can't teach a love for children, and I've always felt a connection to them. You can have the most capable, book-smart teacher, but if they're not genuine, and don't love being with 20 eight-year-olds, that comes through.*

*I love being around 20 to 30 eight-year-olds. It's invigorating. Is that to say I don't think I'd be a good high school teach or coach? No. I think that might be in my future. But I love being around those eight-year-olds. It invigorates me.*

*I'm a much better teacher than when I first started. I thought I was a good teacher my first year, but until you experience a situation you can't prepare for everything. I have become much better at becoming more efficient with my time.*

*Every minute of every day in the NFL was structured. You had somebody telling you what to do, how to do it, when to do it, why to do it. And let's analyze that. In teaching you have to be more of a self-monitoring and self-motivating individual. It's my responsibility to be the pulse and to monitor of how each of my 20 students are doing individually.*

*Having 20 individuals who have up and down days, and being able to figure out if this is this a student who really needs that one-on-one attention today, or if they are just having a bad day because they don't feel good, and being able to manage all those duties that go with being a teacher, and the administration, took some juggling.*

*I now know what being a teacher is really all about, and I'm able to handle it. The more I'm in it, the more I'm glad I made this decision. I just continually love it.*

*Actually, the NFL wasn't drastically harder than teaching. I believe the hours that I put in and the work I do teaching is equivalent to the time and effort I put in when I played football. But you're making one-hundredth of the salary. And that's when I start pondering where our emphasis is in society.*

*I would certainly hope that as a teacher I have a larger impact on these third-grade students' lives than I did as a football player. But at this point, I don't know if I can say that.*

*I mean, that 15 minutes I spent with a child in Indianapolis could be more meaningful than 1,800 hours in the classroom. You don't know what kind of impact you have as a teacher until years later.*

*But if I can make a life-changing impression on even one student, I think that's a successful year.*

AS JAY NEARED the end of his second year as a regular faculty member, anyone who didn't know it would never have guessed that he played pro football for nine seasons. In his classroom, walking the halls and school grounds, or eating lunch at a table with his students, he was that friendly, smiling Mr. Leeuwenburg the boys and girls had come to enjoy so much.

"He's sort of a natural in school life," the Head of School smiles, giving in to his personal feelings just a little. "There's the classroom, but school life is also a lot of casual, informal interactions with kid and parents and adults. We have Lower School assemblies, and he's right in the middle of them. When the kids bring up a volunteer they always grab Jay and make him go up to the front. You better be a good sport in a school setting, and he's a great one.

"When you meet Jay, whatever stereotypes you have about a jock get dissipated in about 10 or 15 minutes. He is counterintuitive to what you think NFL players are like. He's very gentle, very patient in the classroom. He has a very winning personality, very personable, very intelligent. And you need all of those qualities in the classroom.

"I think of him more as a natural classroom teacher than a natural jock. I see his pro career as a byway; otherwise we would have had him in the teaching profession a lot sooner."

An exchange Carole Buschmann had one morning with a colleague at C.A. illustrates how complete Jay's transformation has been.

"When I told one of the teachers I was going to be interviewed for a book about Jay," she related, "that teacher's reaction was, 'Why is someone doing a book about him?'

"When I told her it was about Jay's diabetes and how he became a star in the NFL despite it, she said, 'He WAS?!'

*I try to keep it fairly low-key that I was a professional athlete. Obviously I never deny that I was an NFL player. But I feel like I have so much more to offer these students. I want to show them that I am a teacher; that I am somebody they can learn from.*

*After I've gained their respect and their confidence, I let them into my past life a little bit. But I don't want to be a celebrity; this is not the place for that.*

*It's another story, though, when it comes to parent-teacher conferences. I don't know this for a fact, and I haven't done a survey. But I would say I've had the most* male-attended conferences of anyone in the Lower School.

I was shocked by the number of times the father came with the mother, and the father did most of the talking. Twenty of the 30 minutes of the conference, we talked about CU; we talked about my playing days – 'Oh, I used to live in Chicago . . .'

I'd say, 'You know, you really should talk about little Susie.' And dad would say, 'Oh, I've got no problem with her; she's doing great! Tell me about . . .' At about half the conferences, I felt uncomfortable because we didn't talk about the student.

I have parents tell me, 'You know, so-and-so has an older brother, and he's getting recruited. Can you say something to coach Barnett, because he really wants to go to CU and play football for the Buffs. Do you have any pull?' I don't make any promises.

Every year I have a few students who ask, 'May I have your autograph for my dad?' But I don't want to set up the expectation that if you're in Mr. Leeuwenburg's class, you get an autographed football card.

The last week of school, I bring in all my old helmets and jerseys to school, and the kids can try them on. 'Today's the day.' We can talk football and I'll answer all the questions they have. We'll talk about it for five hours if they want to. But not at start of the year; that would set the wrong emphasis.

I'm not a football player now. I'm their teacher.

# EPILOGUE

LIFE HAS a funny way of bringing people together in situations made for each other. Strangers go off in different directions, unaware the other even exists until, one day, events in their lives unexpectedly converge.

Will Baird was two years old and living in Denver when Jay left Chicago and signed his free agent contract with the Indianapolis Colts. Peter Baird, Will's dad, had cheered Jay as a member of those championship CU Buffs teams and knew he was playing in the NFL, but that's as far as it went. They'd never met.

The next year Will's mom Sue thought her toddler was drinking a lot of water for his age, so she took him to the doctor as a precaution. "Sue had a mother's instinct about Will" her husband says, "and because of that he avoided hospitalization and all of the dramatic stories."

Will was diagnosed with Type 1 diabetes, and came home with one of Jay's life-sized "Yes I Can, Yes You Can" posters. "We put it on his bedroom door as soon as he brought it home,"

Peter says. "It stayed there for years. Will grew up with this man on his door."

As kindergarten approached for Will, the Bairds looked into a few schools. They were looking for individualized instruction, but not specifically thinking about special attention for Will's diabetes. They made application to Colorado Academy, partly because Sue's brother had attended school there. Will was accepted for admission.

By the time Will was finishing second grade, Jay had spent a disappointing season with the Redskins; had thumbed his nose at the Oakland Raiders and told the head coach of the Denver Broncos to go fly a kite; had met Carole Buschman and visited Mesa Verde; and was completing his teaching internship and interviewing for that third grade opening at C.A.

"We were talking with the principal," Peter recalls, "and she said, 'I have great news. We're going to offer Jay the job. And if he takes it, we're going to put Will in his class.' We wanted to tell Will right away that the man on his door was going to be his teacher, but they asked us not to say anything until they knew for sure.

"When it was finally okay for us to tell Will, I said, 'You're not going to believe who your teacher is going to be.' "

*I don't know this to be true, but the way I think of it, it would be almost like reading about a comic book hero, and all of a sudden, he's at your door! You love the idea that he does all these things. But it's not real tangible. Then, it's holy cow! I've seen this guy walking around, and now he's going to be my teacher.*

*The thing I offered Will, as much as anything, was him seeing me live with diabetes every day, and that I was normal. I didn't have this badge that said, 'Look at me, I'm different; look at me, you have to treat me differently.'*

*I was a living example for him, every day, of everything I've talked about: 'This is who I am. It's not all I am, but it's part of my makeup.' I think he felt much more comfortable with the idea of, 'Hmmm, I'm going to take a blood sugar. It's not a big deal.'*

*Will's parents had done such a good job of preparing him that there were times when I saw a young 'me', in that, diabetes-wise, he's very comfortable with his disease. And he was dealing with this earlier than I did.*

*I could help him because I knew what to look for. There were situations that were going on with him, with his blood sugar, that he would not be able to explain to another teacher, but I just knew. He'd be about to go to P.E., and I would say, " Hey, Will. Did you take a blood sugar?" He'd say, "No." I'd say, "Take one."*

*He'd get a number back, a reading, and I'd say, "Well, you need to drink a juice." Or, "You need to take care of this." I'm not saying I did this every time, but it helped reinforce the good habits that were there from his mom and dad.*

*I would also talk about – and this came up many times – characters in books who had diseases, or characters in books who had to take medicines. Or we'd talk about*

*current events, all those things you can kind of tie in.*
*When I would use diabetes as an example, his classmates*
*would say, 'Oh, that's like what Will has, right?' And it*
*wasn't negative; it was just a matter of fact.*

*They thought of Will as different because of his*
*personality and for all the reasons they think everyone is*
*different, not because he has this disease that he has to take*
*insulin or prick his finger for.*

SUE BAIRD knows that Jay made a difference in her son's life, a difference she believes will last a lifetime.

"Will has no self-consciousness about his diabetes," she offered during Will's fourth-grade year, "and he's at an age when kids are self-conscious. He's not embarrassed to do his checks, and he's not embarrassed to get snacks at school when he needs them. He's motivated to take care of himself."

Sue also believes Jay's impact extends far beyond Will.

"Jay raised the awareness level throughout the school," she points out. "In other classes, the teachers would never remind Will about taking his blood sugar, so he didn't do it. Jay would say, 'C'mon Will, we'll do our tests together.' The other kids were jealous.

"They now do things like stock juice and snacks all over the campus. Will used to get funny looks when he told teachers he needed to have those things. They were gracious, but there's a lot more acceptance now."

Jay's greatest influence was on Sue Baird herself, as it

always will be on parents in her situation.

"Here's a guy who has a pretty difficult row to hoe, yet he's so very positive about it," she says with brimming admiration. "He's a great role model for everyone touched by diabetes in any way.

"Other adults I know with diabetes are more reluctant to talk about it. They just keep it to themselves. Instead, Jay always says, 'Let me tell you all about diabetes.' He's always so positive.

"You know, he's even had an impact on me as a parent of a diabetic child. He's made me feel this can be managed. I'm optimistic. He's given me hope."

# Author's Note

MY FATHER developed diabetes late in his life. One of my best friends died of a diabetes-induced heart attack after battling the disease for most of his life. Another friend had one leg amputated at the knee, and came to rely on twice-weekly dialysis to keep him alive.

Yet when I started working with Jay on our book, my knowledge of this demoralizing, potentially deadly disease was next to nothing.

The anguish parents feel when their child is diagnosed; the depression those children face as they try to believe they can live normal, active lives; the burden of a lifetime of daily finger-prick tests and insulin shots; the ignorance and discrimination in schools and on the job; and the life-threatening consequences of failure to manage the disease were all beyond me.

This, I now realize, is the biggest challenge facing the organizations working to raise money to fight diabetes: Diabetes simply does not capture the general public's emotions the way cancer, AIDS and serious public health crises do. Until you experience diabetes first-hand, you are likely to underestimate it as a serious health threat.

It is my hope that Jay's personal triumph over diabetes and his example of determined self-sufficiency – "Yes I Can! Yes You Can!!" – will be a source of motivation and hope to all whose fundamental challenge in life is no different than his.

It is my hope that his willingness to serve as a role model for diabetics of all ages will inspire more people with this disease to become examples for others to follow.

And it is my hope that this book will raise the awareness level of the many who are fortunate enough to have been spared learning the gravity of diabetes the hard way, so they will recognize it for the epidemic it is.

D.D.

# ACKNOWLEDGMENTS

THIS BOOK developed in the spring of 2004 when Denny and two American Diabetes Association representatives met with Jay to discuss the Father of the Year Awards Dinner and his participation as an honoree. Denny left Jay's home that day with one of his "Yes I Can! Yes You Can!" posters, and the belief that the story behind it should be told in all of its entertaining and inspirational detail. In the months that followed we became – in a real way – teammates. Our team ultimately had many players.

Throughout this project our wives, Melanie and Ingher, have been what they always are to us, encouraging, supportive, helpful, unwavering. Their contributions have made this book much better and more complete, in ways only we can fully appreciate. John Temple, editor, president and publisher of the *Rocky Mountain News*, made time to read a draft of the manuscript. His suggestions added depth, and his opinions provided invaluable reinforcement. Dick and Jann Leeuwenburg generously opened their home to a stranger and shared their experiences and private feelings. We thank them for not holding back. Chris Leeuwenburg's vivid recollections enriched several chapters. His enthusiastic cooperation added fuel to our fire.

We owe special thanks to Dr. Pat Wolff, Dale Collier, Gary Barnett, Bill McCartney, Bill Tobin, Carole Buschman, Peter and Sue Baird and Chris Babbs for their willingness to be interviewed for this book; to John McDonough, for his advice, counsel and encouragement from the Bears days to the present; and to Connie Shella, Tom Brodie and Thane Wettig at Eli Lilly, and Don Doumoulin and Sue Thorn Barlow at Roche Diagnostics – without their support the *Yes I Can! Yes You Can!* Poster and Jay's Corner would not have been possible in their ultimate magnitude. We also express our gratitude to the following for the various ways they helped make the book a reality: Karen Brownlee of the Juvenile Diabetes Research Foundation, George Walker and Sue Glass from the Denver office of the American Diabetes Association, Dave Plati, the University of Colorado, Sue Deans, Cliff Grassmick and Neill Woelk of the *The Daily Camera* in Boulder, CO, the *Indianpolis Star* and Dawn Mitchell, the Chicago Bears and Dan Yuska, Leonardo De La Rocha, the staff at Stats, Inc., Kirkwood High School and John Markovick.

The design of this book is a true reflection of the talent and creativity of Scott Johnson, who is Sputnik Design Works. If there is even a comma out of place, it is not the fault of Audrey Friedman Marcus, who meticulously edited the final manuscript. Judy Joseph, founder of Paros Press, is the one who brought them to this work. It has been a true pleasure to collaborate with them.

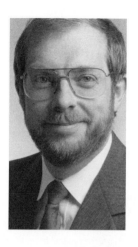

DENNY DRESSMAN is associate managing editor at the *Rocky Mountain News* in Denver, and has been a sports writer and sports editor among his many assignments during a 41-year newspaper career. He previously authored *Gerry Faust: Notre Dame's Man In Motion* and has edited and produced several other books.